T0253840

Essential Concepts of Occupation for Occupational Therapy

Essential Concepts of Occupation for Occupational Therapy is an accessible introduction to vital concepts in occupational science for the occupational therapy practitioner or student. It invites therapists to view and understand their clients differently—by using an "occupational lens" to focus on the lives of their clients as everyday doers. It addresses the key questions at the heart of understanding humans as occupational beings: What do people typically do? And, where, when, how, why, and with whom do they do it?

These questions organize the key concepts from occupational science that form the first chapters of this book, enabling therapists to better understand their clients—and enabling their clients to better understand the importance of occupation to their well-being. Additional chapters clearly describe how therapists can use occupation-based models to apply an expanded view of occupation and make evaluation and intervention more relevant and beneficial to their clients. A final chapter examines trends and lifestyle changes occurring in the 21st century to anticipate how these might impact future practice.

Through use of engaging and thoughtful cases that illustrate many of the concepts, this guide will help practitioners clearly understand their clients as doers, while also providing enhanced ways for therapist to confidently apply these concepts in practice.

Charles Christiansen, Ed.D., OTR, FAOTA, is Professor Emeritus and Former Dean of the School of Health Professions at the University of Texas Medical Branch, and retired CEO of the American Occupational Therapy Foundation.

Kristine Haertl, Ph.D., OTR/L, FAOTA is a Professor in the Department of Occupational Therapy at St. Catherine University. She has extensive publications and presentations on six continents and maintains a private OT practice.

Essential Concepts of Occupation for Occupational Therapy

A Guide to Practice

Charles Christiansen and Kristine Haertl

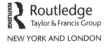
Routledge
Taylor & Francis Group

NEW YORK AND LONDON

Designed cover image: © Getty

First published 2024
by Routledge
605 Third Avenue, New York, NY 10158

and by Routledge
4 Park Square, Milton Park, Abingdon, Oxon, OX14 4RN

Routledge is an imprint of the Taylor & Francis Group, an informa business

Library of Congress Cataloging-in-Publication Data
A catalog record for this title has been requested

ISBN: 9781032150307 (hbk)
ISBN: 9781032150291 (pbk)
ISBN: 9781003242185 (ebk)

DOI: 10.4324/9781003242185

Typeset in Times New Roman
by Deanta Global Publishing Services, Chennai, India

This book is dedicated to our colleagues Elizabeth Yerxa, Gary Kielhofner, Gail Fidler, Mary Reilly, and Ann Wilcock. During their professional lives as scholars, they were committed to ensuring that the ardent study and therapeutic use of *occupation* would never be relegated to footnotes in accounts of occupational therapy's history. Their commitment lives on.

Contents

Foreword

Elizabeth Townsend

Essential Concepts of Occupation for Occupational Therapy is a beautifully written, well-organized book that, in ten chapters, builds on the growing range of publications worldwide for those eager to know more about *doing* or everyday activity and engagement—expressed here in English as "occupation" in line with the profession, *occupational* therapy, and the scholarly focus of *occupational* science.

What humans *do* each day in different times, places, cultures, and communities has long been recognized as a foundation of human existence. What we do determines food, shelter, and safety combined with what we aspire to do for happiness, health, and freedoms in societies, in communities and our individual lives. *Essential Concepts of Occupation* for Occupational Therapy takes a refreshing look at what humans do beyond this taken-for-granted awareness of occupation. Christiansen and Haertl stimulate deep thinking about occupation with interesting insights on occupation, including historical recognition of the term in English speaking countries. They consider: the importance of meaningful occupation; identity through occupation; personality theory and occupation; occupation embedded in and defining time use and place; cultural issues and occupation; justice foundations in occupation; occupation-based theory; occupation-based evaluation; occupation-based intervention; and human occupation in the future.

Readers may want to translate or substitute the "concepts of occupation" using terms such as daily activities, human capabilities, community resources, family life, social issues, equity, justice, especially outside Western cultures. The Western focus on individualism is to be expected, given the individualized organization and funding of health services where occupational therapists in the Northern, Western parts of the world are best known for now.

Christiansen opens the book with four chapters drawing on his expertise in the North American–European history of occupational therapy, connections between American occupational therapy and occupational science, connections between occupation, identity, and meaning, and connections between time, place, and occupation—in what people do.

Chapter 1 offers an excellent summary of the history of explicit recognition that occupation is associated with health. As Christiansen states, the organization of services using work as an activity cure emerged in 19th-century England and France with the naming of a therapy of occupation, now known as occupational therapy. He argues that there has been strength in the reciprocal relationship of occupational therapy since the 1980s with the scholarly field of occupational science. In Chapter 2, Christiansen advances the important argument that meaningful occupation in daily life is a necessary element to examine when looking at health, well-being, and justice. His research provides evidence of the positive impacts of participation in occupation as well as the problematic restrictions in participation for some populations and individuals. Christiansen continues in Chapter 3 with research that connects personality traits with occupation, showing how interests and preferences for activity are organized using personality theory. From the world of work, referring to officially recognized occupations, Christiansen quotes John Holland's theory of six occupational types (Doer, Thinker, Creator, Helper, Organizer, and Persuader), categories used to organize job classifications and wages by the United States Department of Labor as reflected on the official O*Net website. Furthermore, he highlights research on personality theory and personal narrative as a window to personal meaning. Chapter 4 profiles Christiansen's long-held interest to examine how time and place influence what people do. He points to the importance of time use data collected for populations as the basis to understand social trends and economics; his research on individual occupations refers to biological factors, such as circadian rhythms, that influence rest activity cycles, which in turn affect energy, attention, and sleep. Research on place differentiates between archetypal places, associated with occupations or activities (such as kitchens and bathrooms), and natural or symbolic places that invite certain occupations or activities (such as places of worship).

The next four chapters by Haertl flow nicely from the first four, profiling her expertise in the relationship between occupation and culture, her interests in social and occupational justice, her knowledge of occupation-based theories and occupational therapy practice models, and her expertise in occupation-based evaluation.

Chapter 5 presents important research on how families and social groups influence occupational choice and engagement throughout the lifespan. Haertl highlights the concept of co-occupation to show how simultaneous participation influences the occupational engagement of multiple persons. She discusses how the environment impacts individual and group participation in occupation. To emphasize sociocultural influences on occupation, Haertl raises attention to human life occurring in multiple cultural groups, each cultural context uniquely influencing occupational choice and participation. In Chapter 6, Haertl takes on the complex yet essential connections that can be seen when occupation is viewed from a social justice lens. She presents a current definition of occupational justice and commonly (to date) described forms of occupational injustice, each of which speaks to violations of human rights (occupational rights). She offers a very helpful discussion of some key conditions of occupational injustice, including underemployment and unemployment, institutionalization, and displacement. Readers will learn about working with the Participatory Occupational Justice Framework (POJF) at the individual, systems, or population levels. Chapter 7 offers a very practical overview of American and other Western occupation-based theories and practice models. Haertl acknowledges that the theories and models she presents are largely relevant for working with individuals. She emphasizes the idea of goodness-of-fit referring to the importance of congruence between the person, contextual factors, and occupation; and she presents occupation as both a means—a tool—to use in occupational therapy practices, and the end outcome defined typically as occupational performance. Chapter 8 provides an essential introduction to occupation-based evaluation. She defines this as evaluation that examines occupation at the core. The ideal is to evaluate actual performance of tasks, using top-down approaches that put a spotlight on occupational outcomes and processes, differentiating this from evaluating strength or cognition as components of occupations. Haertl concludes by emphasizing the importance in occupation-based evaluation of the environment to understand the context for occupational engagement.

The final two chapters introduce occupation-based intervention and reflect on human occupation in the future. In Chapter 9 Haertl emphasizes the opportunities for occupational therapists to use occupation-focused and occupation-based interventions that have meaning for individuals, families, and groups in the cultural, social, and economic environments where people live, play, and work. Chapter 10 presents a fascinating Capstone as Christiansen knits the book together with reflections on human occupation in the future. Work and all our occupations are changing because of climate change, advancing digital technologies, geopolitical tensions, pandemics, and social unrest. We may be witnessing the fourth industrial revolution with automation, artificial intelligence (AI), and robotics. Humans are already facing rapid technological changes, unemployment, loneliness, and distrust of public institutions. These and other social conditions are resulting in mental illnesses such as depression, substance use, anxiety, and aggression toward others.

The book ends by emphasizing the growing need for occupational therapists—an exponential, urgent growth in need for more occupational therapists and occupational scientists around the world given current and changing conditions. May you enjoy and use this "Practitioner's Guide' emerging from the scholarly partnership of Charles Christiansen and Kristine Haertl.

Elizabeth Townsend, PhD
Dalhousie University, Nova Scotia, Canada
April 2023

Preface

This book is aimed at introducing the reader to major concepts of occupational science and their application to occupational therapy practice. The study of occupation (occupational science) and the application of knowledge about occupation to health and well-being (occupational therapy) are naturally connected. Each can complement the other.

Understanding everyday living seems straightforward at first thought. But behind nearly every daily action and interaction there are numerous factors that help explain *what, why, when, where,* and *how* occupations occur. This book is an introduction to those factors and how they can be better understood and used effectively to address the many challenges of living associated with health and well-being.

The study of occupation is complex, but with the right perspective, it becomes easier. For over a century, people with great minds, humanitarian values, and commitment from many fields have contributed insights and research toward understanding people as doers. No claim is made that this book is an authoritative summary of that work. Instead, the aim has been to select information that may genuinely enhance the perspectives of therapists in their understanding of clients as occupational beings. Life is a laboratory for understanding occupation; and what is learned can often be applied toward better understanding oneself.

The reader can be better prepared for reading and understanding the chapters in this book by considering these recommendations:

1. *Having an occupational perspective is* essential. This means observing people doing everyday activities (occupations) in the world through the lens of *doing.* One should always ask, what conditions or influences might help explain *what, when, where, how,* or *why* an observed activity is being done?
2. *Occupational therapy uses a biopsychosocial perspective.* That means it does not focus on the biological causes of a condition, but rather emphasizes how multiple interacting domains (biological, psychological, and

social) influence health and a person's ability to accomplish tasks that are necessary or important.

3. *A complete understanding of health goes beyond the body and mind to include the social environment.* This means that places and people are an important part of the client's everyday setting. People flourish through their relationships with others, by residing safely and harmoniously in groups, and by having access to basic resources necessary for pursuing their lives. This illustrates why social determinants of health and well-being are very important to occupational therapists. These ideas underlie the World Health Organization (WHO) definition of health:

    "Health is a state of complete physical, mental and social well-being and not merely the absence of disease or infirmity." In this book, well-being is defined as *a positive state that includes a person's state of health and satisfaction with their current life situation.*

4. The occupational therapy process is *client-centered* and has three parts: *Evaluation, Intervention,* and *Outcomes.* It can provide services to individual clients, groups, or populations and is always focused on *occupational engagement.* A key part of evaluation is the *occupational profile,* providing information on the client from an occupational perspective.

5. *A useful understanding of a client generally requires some narrative reasoning.* This means that the therapy provider tries to understand the client's current situation in the overall context of the client's life story.

The authors have intended to provide a useful and current resource aimed at students early in their studies. Wherever possible, the latest published information has been cited to support information. Yet, the years ahead will be characterized by transformative change. This makes it especially important for readers to adopt a practice philosophy that is flexible and well informed. Hopefully the perspectives shared above will be sufficiently timeless to be useful, regardless of what the future brings.

Although this is a co-authored book, each author assumed a role as lead author for specific chapters. Dr. Christiansen assumed this role for Chapters 1 through 4, and Chapter 10. Dr. Haertl served as lead author for Chapters 5 through 9.

Finally, and importantly, the authors gratefully acknowledge the generous assistance of Drs. Elizabeth Townsend, Hannah Oldenburg, Ashlea Cardin, and Paula Rabaey. We are also indebted to others who consented to be in photographs used to exemplify points in the book.

Chapter 1

Occupational Science and Its Relationship to Occupational Therapy

Introduction

Humans are **occupational beings**. This statement might seem strange to most people, but it is an important and fundamental truth. Humans exist with a built-in drive to explore and act on the world. In other words, they are innate *doers* (White, 1959). Understanding this innate drive and its complexity is the subject of this book. Specifically, this book was written to explain how knowledge about human occupation can be used to advantage in the practice of **occupational therapy**.

Over the years, multiple definitions have been offered by scholars to clarify the **meaning** of occupation, each with variations. The word **occupation** stems from a Latin term meaning to *seize* or *occupy*. Occupation is activity that seizes the interest and attention of people, and thus occupies their time.

A founder of occupational therapy and physician, William Rush Dunton, once wrote that occupation is "a basic human need as essential as food, drink and the air we breathe" (Dunton, 1919). The founders of **occupational science** (the study of occupation) defined occupation in a quaint way as "chunks of culturally and personally meaningful activity in which humans engage that can be named in the lexicon [vocabulary] of [the] culture" (Clark et al. 1991, p. 301). Other definitions of occupation are identified in Box 1.1, and a quick review shows that the definitions share common elements; namely that occupations involve humans *doing* intentional everyday activities that are *meaningful* to them.

DOI: 10.4324/9781003242185-1

BOX 1.1 DEFINING OCCUPATION

Selected definitions of occupation from different organizations reveal similar perspectives

- "Groups of activities and tasks of everyday life, named, organized, and given value and meaning by individuals and a culture; everything people do to occupy themselves, including looking after themselves (self-care), enjoying life (leisure) and contributing to the social and economic fabric of their communities (productivity)" (Canadian Association of Occupational Therapists, 2008, pp. 24–25).
- "Everyday personalized activities that people do as individuals, in families, and with communities to occupy time and bring meaning and purpose to life. Occupations can involve the execution of multiple activities for completion and can result in various outcomes. The broad range of occupations is categorized as activities of daily living, instrumental activities of daily living, health management, rest and sleep, education, work, play, leisure, and social participation" (American Occupational Therapy Association, 2020, p. 79).
- "Occupations refer to the everyday activities that people do as individuals, in families and with communities to occupy time and bring meaning and purpose to life. Occupations include things people need to, want to and are expected to do" (World Federation of Occupational Therapy, 2022).

It is thus understandable that occupational therapy scholars identify humans as "occupational beings," a singular way of saying that people have a natural drive to do the things that are necessary for their existence and enjoyment (White, 1971). Indeed, for all group-living animals, survival depends on *doing things*, whether seeking shelter, avoiding danger, or finding food and water.

The simple phrase "doing things" immediately reveals the two-sided nature of occupation. On the one side, it involves the *act* or *action* of doing. But doing what? For humans and other animals, the act of doing has a purpose, and what is done or completed becomes that purpose enacted. The occupational therapy scholar David Nelson was among the first to examine and describe this two-sided nature of occupation. He used the terms *form* and *performance* to explain the two dimensions implied by the simple phrase "doing things." In Nelson's explanation, the word form described the "thing" that was being done (like eating, or reading, or playing); while the word performance was used to describe the doing or active part of occupation (Nelson, 1988).

Occupational Engagement

The term **occupational engagement** is often used to describe humans doing purposeful activities that are meaningful to them (Yerxa, 1980; Wilcock, 2006, pp. 315–316). There are differences and inconsistencies in how the term occupational engagement is defined or used in the occupational therapy literature and understood in practice. However, there is general agreement that occupational engagement means more than simply "an act of doing something" (Black, et al., 2019; Kennedy & Davis, 2017; Cruz et al., 2023). It seems that occupational engagement does not require physical performance but does require the personal involvement of an individual in a manner that involves their interest, attention, and purpose. Together, these characteristics imply that when people are *engaged* in purposeful occupation, their involvement has meaning to them.

In this book, occupational engagement is not considered a synonym for **participation**. For example, everyday routines, such as grooming or driving, are often performed automatically without much thought or attention directed toward the activity. People often "participate" in meetings (or religious services), yet may be focused on other matters. The detached or automatic performance of certain recurring occupations will be discussed more fully in a later chapter. The point is that there may be different reasons for why people are not fully engaged when they are doing things. They may be distracted, bored, tired, disinterested, or daydreaming. But if they are mostly not attending to their activity, regardless of how important it may be, they are not occupationally engaged. It is possible (perhaps likely) that within the span of time that may be devoted to a given goal-oriented task, people's level of engagement will vary. This would make for interesting research, since there are many aspects of occupation that remain unstudied, and many assumptions that have gone unchallenged (e.g. Hammell, 2009).

Beginning with its founding 70 years earlier, teachers and therapists in occupational therapy have grappled with defining occupation. Yet they agreed that there was a *what* and *how* and *why* for every task. But the focus then was on the therapeutic uses of activity, and not *what*, *why*, and *how* people pursued activities in their everyday lives.

That changed in the late 1980s as specialized graduate study in human occupation began with the aim of answering such questions—with a particular interest in how everyday activities influenced health (Yerxa et al., 1989).

Occupation, Occupational Therapy, and Occupational Science

Historians have traced the origins of occupational therapy to social movements in the 19th century (Christiansen, 2021; Christiansen & Haertl, 2018), and even before that, to certain ideas, such as the moral and humane care for mental illness that began to evolve in Europe (Bing, 1981). The use of purposeful activities to engage mental patients living in "asylums" was a significant development (Anderson & Reed, 2017); but other events helped to give the idea of "occupation" as a curative or healing agent additional momentum.

The Work Cure

In the 19th century, the quality of medical care varied greatly, and practitioners ranged from those who completed training in "storefront" apprenticeships to more in-depth courses of study in colleges and universities. Although the oldest university-based medical school in the United States dates to 1765 (Geiger, 2014) the few established academic medical programs in 1917 were insufficient redundant to produce the number of doctors needed for that era. Medical research was just getting started. As result, medical and surgical care had limited options to address serious injuries and disease, making it necessary to rely on the human body's remarkable ability to heal itself as a primary approach to treatment. Often, the prescription for illness was rest, and occasionally, this **rest cure** was augmented by "the water cure," which consisted of spending curative time relaxing and bathing in natural springs, or near oceans. The water cure approach dated to prehistoric times and was based on the idea that the minerals and warmth of water promoted healing (Rutkow, 2012). Such **water cure** settings, or spas, were popular healing destinations throughout the world, but especially in Europe and Japan (Van Tubergen & Van Der Linden, 2002). The water cure often involved a bathing regimen combined with diet and exercise that was prescribed carefully according to the established practices of each location.

A third type of "cure" that became popular was the **work cure**, a shorthand for prescribing purposeful activities to help people remain active during convalescence and focus on thoughts other than their illnesses. When used in mental asylums, this approach sometimes included participation in productive work tasks such as maintenance, gardening, housekeeping, or cooking; or it might involve various non-work pursuits fostering rest and relaxation (Reed, 2005). For wealthier patients, small specialized private hospitals focused on arts and crafts, leisure, and recreation (Anthony, 2005).

The implication here was that there was a connection between the mind and body that was important to the healing process. The use of arts and crafts that emphasized functional design, a connection to nature, and hand-crafted authenticity was an offshoot of this idea that had gained wide social popularity at the time because of its claimed connection to moral fitness and health (Levine, 1987). This was an important development, because for years medicine had been operating with the false belief that there was no connection between the mind and body. This was called **mind–body dualism** and can be traced to French philosopher René Descartes (Henk & Ten Have, 1987; see Figure 1.1).

Support for the ideas behind the work cure was given additional momentum by Romanticism, a way of thinking about life that included ideas such as self-reliance, craftsmanship, social justice, and the celebration of art and nature. This movement

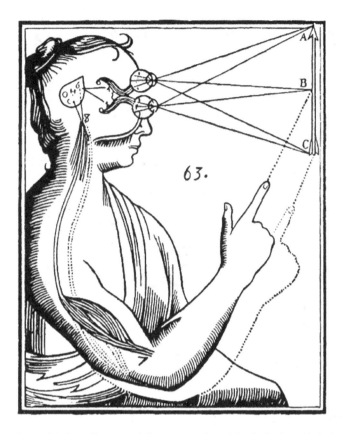

Figure 1.1 René Descartes' illustration of mind–body dualism. He believed that sensations
were passed to the brain and from there to the immaterial spirit (this media
file is in the public domain)

created a favorable social attitude toward the idea that human activity could be
seen as restorative (Christiansen, 2021). The application of the work cure in mental
asylums was a natural extension of these ideas and provided favorable conditions
for the founding of the occupational therapy profession (Luchins, 1988).

Public Support for Humane Care in Asylums

Clifford Whittingham Beers, an educated and affluent mental patient who
spent time in several of America's facilities for the mentally ill, became a popular national advocate for the reform of large mental institutions. His popular
book, *A Mind that Found Itself* (Beers, 1908), described his mistreatment by
staff in the facilities where he was being treated. This motivated reform efforts,
including the creation of societies to promote mental health and prevent mental

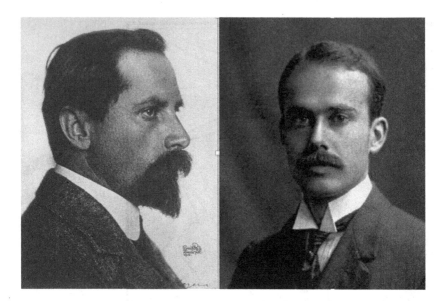

Figure 1.2 Adolf Meyer [L] and Clifford Whittingham Beers [R] worked together to improve conditions in mental asylums, thus supporting the founding and evolution of occupational therapy and the mental hygiene movement (Meyer: Camill Ruf (1872–1939)—IHM, public domain; Beers: Public domain, Wikimedia Commons)

illness—collectively called the **mental hygiene movement** (Parry, 2010). Beers worked closely with a prominent psychiatrist of the day, Adolf Meyer, who believed that reforms should include new hospitals having workshops for occupations. Meyer had been influenced by Eleanor Clarke Slagle and by his visits to an immigrant settlement community in Chicago known as Hull House, where Slagle had trained (Christiansen, 2007; see Figure 1.2).

Origins of Occupational Science

Earlier, occupational science was best defined as a discipline dedicated to the study of humans as *doers*. As such, it draws from other disciplines studying human behavior. Historians agree that occupational science originated at the University of Southern California, which established the first doctoral program in the discipline in 1989 (Anderson & Reed, 2017, p. 257). The purpose of the program was to advance research and study to better understand human occupation and its complexities, and to provide a solid scientific basis for occupational therapy practice (Yerxa et al., 1989).

The importance of this new science became apparent over the following decade. By the early 21st century, the field of occupational science had organized a research society, a scientific journal, and programs of study at several colleges and universities in the United States and other countries (Clark, 2006). Today, those programs continue to evolve, and a growing body of research has revealed useful insights into the astonishing complexity of human occupation.

In this book, readers will learn that although human occupation may seem simple (after all, it's how people spend their time), it has many layers of complexity. *What motivates people to choose one activity over another? When and how do people do what they do? What pursuits are engaging and meaningful to them?* These are just some of the many questions that are relevant to fully understanding occupation, and questions of this type form the basis for some of the research that is done by occupational scientists.

The Relationship between Occupational Science and Occupational Therapy

Most fields of human endeavor begin with understanding aspects of the world through observation and study. Galileo, Newton, Hippocrates, and others were curious about the world around them. Their basic discoveries encouraged like-minded individuals to further pursue the basic sciences of biology, physics, and chemistry. Others applied knowledge from these fields to create solutions to the practical needs of society (like engineering, architecture, and medicine). Because these fields apply knowledge from the basic sciences, they are called **applied sciences**.

Yet, occupational therapy (another applied science) drew its early knowledge mostly from other applied fields in the life sciences, such as psychology, anthropology, sociology, and medicine, because occupational science had not yet been established. Yet, in the 1980s, something changed. Mary Reilly (1963), a scholar at the University of Southern California, encouraged her graduate students to explore a framework for understanding occupational behavior. Later, Kielhofner and colleagues (e.g., Kielhofner & Burke, 1980) proposed an elaborate model of human occupation to serve as a basis for practice that would supplant "the **medical model**" that had influenced practice for several decades. A resurgence of interest in human occupation by occupational therapy scholars seemed to take root, and this led to the emergence of occupational science.

The rationale was that if human occupation was to be the basis for occupational therapy practice, a more in-depth, scientifically based understanding of occupation would be necessary (Yerxa et al., 1989).

The Push for Evidence

It is true that when occupational therapy was founded, it used occupation as a basis for therapy before much (if any) research had been done to demonstrate and understand how it worked. Instead, the founders and early occupational therapists used common sense and experience to guide their work, and this proved to be sufficient and acceptable during most of occupational therapy's first century.

Other health-related fields, including medicine, also based much of their early practice on experience and common sense as well.

Then, in the 1990s, a broad societal push for **evidence-based practice** began (Sackett et al., 1996). Evidence-based practice refers specifically to approaches in health care that are supported by rigorous research. Although the profession's need for research to support practice had been recognized much earlier (Christiansen, 1983; West, 1981), the number of qualified researchers was limited. By the start of the millennium, there were sufficient scholars available to respond to calls for more evidence to support practice (Tickle-Degnen, 2000). This led to targeted grant programs by the federal government and the American Occupational Therapy Foundation as well as dramatic growth in the publication of research (Classen, 2018).

Evidence-based Practice and Occupation-based Therapy

The movement toward evidence-based practice in occupational therapy often encouraged research that focused more on specific interventions and procedures than on research that explored the basic nature of human occupation and its relationship to **well-being**. The use of terms such as *occupation-focused* or *occupation-based* to describe interventions clearly implies that some occupational therapy is not based on occupation. This has reopened a profession-wide discussion on what types of therapy are truly *occupational* in the sense originally embraced by the profession (Fisher, 2014).

The Means and End of Occupation

In a century-old field with a distinguished history of recognizing occupation as a unique approach to healing, it might seem extraordinary to question the value of using occupation as an approach to treatment. Yet, some occupational therapists believe that any therapy is occupational if its aim is to enable or restore a person's ability to engage in meaningful occupations. In this sense, occupation is viewed as an end, or the outcome of an intervention. Proponents of this perspective seem to argue that the end justifies the means, claiming that the way the outcome is achieved is less important than the result that is accomplished.

Others hold the view that *authentic* occupational therapy requires the use of meaningful occupation as a central feature of intervention (Yerxa, 1967). They argue that the value of therapy resides in the process of *doing*, especially where the activity is chosen by the client and the purpose is meaningful to the client. This represents a view of occupation as therapeutic *means*. This perspective claims that occupation as means involves another very important feature that influences therapeutic outcomes. This is the personal meaning of the occupation to the client.

Tailored versus Standardized Interventions

In today's evidence-based practice, the trend in many places favors interventions that are standardized so that they can be studied and validated across clients. **Standardized interventions** use protocols and manuals that carefully describe how interventions should be done. In contrast, **tailored interventions** are those that are individually chosen or modified for the personal characteristics of an individual patient or client (Richards et al., 2007). In early occupational therapy, an effort was made to customize therapy to the characteristics and personality of the client. However, tailored interventions represent a modification of those earlier approaches, in that tailored intervention typically refers to a given intervention customized to the client, rather than the use of a different type of intervention altogether, which was common in occupational therapy in earlier years.

Does this mean that manualized (standardized) therapy is less effective? And is this question relevant to *occupational therapy* or *occupational science*? Perhaps this represents an opportunity to ask a general question about whether personalized, meaningful approaches influence an individual's overall performance and satisfaction with therapy?

The authors of this book propose that questions about *how* an individual's personal characteristics and life circumstances influence their occupational choices and performance are relevant to both occupational therapy and occupational science. In occupational therapy, the various influences on people doing occupations during their everyday lives can be relevant to the **occupational profile** of a client being served by an occupational therapist.

The Occupational Profile

Occupational profile is a term used in occupational therapy to describe collective information gathered on a client's occupational history, interests, and skills. This profile includes an overview of the client's narrative, or life story, especially where such information is relevant to understanding the client, the client's condition, and intervention possibilities. It is widely accepted that connecting interventions to the lives of clients helps individualize treatment, gives interventions relevance and meaning, and helps engage clients in the therapeutic process (Hammell, 2004). Further chapters in this book provide additional information about the nature and value of creating an occupational profile for each client receiving occupational therapy.

Connecting Occupational Therapy and Occupational Science

Occupational science evolved from an idea that occupational therapy needs occupational science to provide the foundational knowledge necessary for guiding its practice. Yet, the relationship is also reciprocal because information from therapists can be useful to occupational scientists. Scholars in occupational science view knowledge that *includes* studies of the application of occupation in occupational therapy practice as relevant to their work (Society for the Study of Occupation, 2019). In this book, the authors agree with the viewpoint that occupational therapy and occupational science are complementary in nature. This means that they augment and strengthen each other and differ mainly in their respective areas of focus.

The areas of interest for occupational science include any matters related to how humans purposely use time in their daily lives. The areas of interest to occupational therapists include information about occupations that are relevant to interventions that enable performance and participation in life. These areas clearly overlap, and it is this area of common interest that best describes how occupational therapy and occupational science complement each other.

What Occupations are Relevant to Occupational Therapy?

Adolf Meyer, the prominent psychiatrist and early advocate of occupational therapy, believed strongly that the lives of his patients were closely connected to their illnesses, and that part of the healing process should involve a normalization of their daily activities. He observed that healthy routines included a balance of work, rest, and play (Meyer, 1922) and thus became one of the first scholars to identify areas of occupation relevant to practice. But it was not until decades later that occupational therapy began to name, define, and classify these areas for scholarly purposes (Christiansen, 1994). Today, the domains of human occupation identified by the American Occupational Therapy Association include *work, play, leisure, education, rest and sleep, health management, activities of daily living, instrumental activities of daily living*, and *social participation* (American Occupational Therapy Association, 2020, p. 35; see Table 1.1).

Clearly, these categories are not intended to be mutually exclusive since they overlap. For example, social participation often occurs during meals (an activity of daily living), play, leisure, and education; just as health management may include rest and sleep or shopping (an instrumental activity of daily living) for medications and supplies. The primary purpose of these categories is to provide convenient groupings for organizing and describing them rather than for their use in scientific research. The groupings are sometimes associated with the locations or places where these categories of occupations are performed. Sleep and many ADL occupations (such as dressing, bathing, grooming) are typically done inside the client's place of living (e.g., the bathroom or bedroom). In contrast, many instrumental activities of daily living (such as shopping, religious expression, and driving) take place away from a personal residence.

International time use scientists gathering data for economic forecasting and social trends have accepted the challenge of finding standardized categories of

Table 1.1 Categories of occupation in occupational therapy and their descriptions

Activities of daily living	Routine activities to take care of one's body such as bathing, toileting, dressing, meal preparation, grooming, sexual activity, and necessary daily living movement within one's habitat.
Instrumental activities of daily living	Caring for children, others, including pets; communicating; moving around a community; shopping; managing finances, meal preparation and cleanup; home management; spiritual expression.
Health management	Managing medications, symptoms, nutrition, activity, equipment, emotions, and interactions with providers and organizations.
Rest and sleep	Relaxing to restore energy, preparing self and one's environment for sleep, sustaining a sleep state.
Education	Investigating, selecting, and participating in vocational, academic, and extracurricular activities to enhance knowledge, information, and skills.
Work	Exploring opportunities, and seeking, acquiring; and maintaining paid or unpaid activities related to one's goals and interests.
Play	Participating in activities that are intrinsically motivated and freely chosen.
Leisure	Participating in activities that are not obligatory and done in one's discretionary time.
Social participation	Interacting with peers, partners, family, friends, or others in a group or community.

Source: Charles Christiansen. Adapted from descriptions provided from various sources by AOTA (2020).

daily human activity. These scientists have collaboratively identified methods for minimizing differences in time use classification systems to make their studies more internationally comparable and to increase their accuracy (Vikat & Boko, 2013). These classifications are identified and discussed in Chapter 4.

Expanding the Scope of Understanding and Practice

In the not-so-distant past, the scope of occupational therapy practice omitted occupations such as smoking, sleep, or sex (Anderson & Reed, 2017). These omissions generally went unquestioned. Yet, in today's broader understanding of lifestyles and health, it seems shortsighted to exclude any domain of human occupation as irrelevant, no matter how socially controversial it might seem. The value of understanding occupations viewed as controversial, unhealthy, or "socially deviant" is now supported both in occupational therapy practice and in occupational science (Kiepek et al., 2019; Twinley, 2021).

The recognition that lifestyles influence health and well-being, and the prevalence of therapists in positions that serve communities and populations have expanded the field's views about relevant domains of practice. There are now therapists who work in prisons, homeless facilities, shelters for abused women, refugee camps, and addiction treatment centers, and this list is steadily increasing, again reflecting the growing awareness that health is largely connected to and determined by social factors, which include everyday routines, occupational choices, and lifestyles (Marmot & Wilkinson, 2005).

Occupation as a Cornerstone of Occupational Therapy

Regardless of where occupational therapists practice, there are four cornerstones or foundational characteristics that are viewed as making the profession distinct. These cornerstones are currently identified by the American Occupational Therapy Association as:

- Core values and beliefs rooted in occupation.
- Knowledge of and expertise in the therapeutic use of occupation.
- Professional behaviors and dispositions.
- Therapeutic use of self.

These distinct foundations of practice are supported by several other values and commitments, which include (among others) professional ethics, practice competence, evidence-based and client-centered care, cultural awareness, lifelong learning, and client advocacy (American Occupational Therapy Association, 2020). Yet, earlier versions of the practice framework have identified *basic knowledge about occupation* (and not just therapeutic occupation) as important foundations to practice (e.g., see Gutman et al., 2007). The authors strongly believe that knowledge of certain basic concepts about human occupation *is essential to informed and competent practice.*

What Occupational Therapists Should Know about Occupation

The case supporting the vital connection between occupation and occupational therapy leads to an important question, and one that is central to the purpose of this book: *What basic knowledge about occupation do occupational therapists need to know?* Some scholars in the profession might suggest that the answer to this question depends on the area of practice in which the therapist is practicing. Others might say that some basic knowledge about occupation and how it is related to health and wellness is essential, regardless of an occupational therapist's area of practice.

Consensus Views of Knowledge Required about Occupation

A 21st-century international consensus study of scholars in occupational science (most of whom were also occupational therapists) attempted to answer this question (Backman, et al., 2021). These experts, working independently across three groups, identified 11 consensus concepts about occupation that were seen as essential knowledge for beginning occupational therapy practitioners. The scope of each concept was defined by the experts using a series of consensus-building rounds known as the Delphi method. Although the specific definitions of each area are too extensive to include here, the concept labels from the study are listed below in order of strength of agreement, followed by a summary of the content included in each concept.

1. *Occupation and wellness, health, and well-being.* A general knowledge of the relationship between occupations and wellness, health, and well-being.
2. *The social, cultural, and institutional contexts of occupation.* How relationships, cultural influences, and organizations influence what, when, how, and why people engage in occupations.
3. *Occupation as the core of occupational science and occupational therapy.* How knowledge of occupation is central to people's lives and how it can be used in a therapeutic manner.
4. *Occupational justice.* How social, cultural, and organizational factors create injustices that restrict access to participation and thus can have health consequences.
5. *Occupational meaning.* How occupations organize experiences and help people make sense of their lives.
6. *Occupation and identity.* How current and past experiences provide a framework for describing how people are understood by themselves and others.
7. *The experience of doing occupation.* The sensations and feelings from doing occupation that can enable a sense of existence and satisfaction.
8. *Habits, routines, and patterns of occupation.* The organized and repeated actions and processes that describe occupation and enable their purposes to be met.
9. *The temporal nature of occupation.* The factors that influence the timing, duration, and frequency of occupation.
10. *Occupational balance and imbalance.* The lifestyle factors (nature, frequency, and duration of occupational engagement) that can lead to positive or negative consequences.
11. *The spatial context of occupation.* How the place or setting where occupations are done influences how they are performed and experienced.

These concepts, and a few others, are central to the organization of this book. Thus, the next chapter discusses the relationships between occupation and health, followed by a chapter examining how occupations influence personal meaning and **identity**. The question of how time and place influence what people do forms the basis for Chapter 4. Chapter 5 then addresses how social influences, such as expectations, customs, and relationships, influence what people do and where, and when they engage in certain occupations. These lead to a discussion in Chapter 6 of the social conditions that impede or restrict participation, the health consequences of such social conditions and inequities, and the injustices that these consequences expose. This area of discussion is described broadly in both the occupational science and occupational therapy literature under the term "occupational justice," which implies a belief that engagement in meaningful occupation is imperative for health and well-being across individuals, groups, and populations (Townsend & Wilcock, 2004).

The final chapters of this book deal with the application of occupation in the therapeutic process, including chapters on occupation-based models and frameworks, occupation-based evaluation, and occupation-based approaches to intervention. The book concludes with a chapter on occupations of the future, discussing how current trends in human occupation, including work, leisure, and self-care, might intersect with global changes in climate, migration, and technology, to influence the nature of health care, lifestyles, and occupational therapy practice with individuals, groups, and populations in the future.

Collectively, the overall goal of the chapters in this book is to provide an overview of basic concepts about human occupation to help readers better appreciate its complexity and understand why it serves as an important foundational cornerstone for occupational therapy practice.

BOX 1.2 THE POINT IS:

- The use of occupation as a means for restoring health emerged in the 19th century as the "work cure" and was a precursor to the development of occupational therapy as a profession.
- Occupational science began in the 1980s as a discipline to study humans as doers, and to serve as a basis for advancing knowledge for occupation-based therapy.
- Knowledge of and expertise in the therapeutic use of occupation is one of four cornerstones of occupational therapy practice. This expertise is strengthened by knowledge about human occupation from occupational science.
- Occupational therapy and occupational science are complementary. Knowledge from occupational science enhances practice, and the observations about the use of occupation-based interventions in practice is valuable to occupational scientists.

References

American Occupational Therapy Association. (2020). Occupational therapy practice framework: Domain and process (4th ed.). *American Journal of Occupational Therapy*, 74 (Suppl. 2), 7412410010. https://doi.org/10.5014/ajot.2020.74S2001

Anderson, L., & Reed, K. L. (2017). *The history of occupational therapy: The first century*. Slack.

Anthony, S. H. (2005). Dr. Herbert J. Hall: Originator of honest work for occupational therapy 1904–1923 [Part I]. *Occupational Therapy in Health Care, 19*(3), 3–19.

Backman, C. L., Christiansen, C. H., Hooper, B. R., Pierce, D., & Price, M. P. (2021). Occupational science concepts essential to occupation-based practice: Development of expert consensus. *The American Journal of Occupational Therapy*, 75(6), 7506205120. https://doi.org/10.5014/ajot.2021.049090

Beers, C. W. (1908). *A mind that found itself*. Longmans, Green.

Bing, R. K. (1981). Occupational therapy revisited: A paraphrastic journey. *The American Journal of Occupational Therapy*, 35(8), 499–518.

Black, M. H., Milbourn, B., Desjardins, K., Sylvester, V., Parrant, K., & Buchanan, A. (2019). Understanding the meaning and use of occupational engagement: Findings from a scoping review. *British Journal of Occupational Therapy*, 82(5), 272–287.

Canadian Association of Occupational Therapists. (2008). CAOT position statement: Occupations and health. *Occupational Therapy Now, 11*(1), 24–26.

Christiansen, C. H. (1983). Research: An economic imperative. *The Occupational Therapy Journal of Research*, 3(4), 195–198.

Christiansen, C. (1994). Classification and study in occupation a review and discussion of taxonomies. *Journal of Occupational Science, 1*(3), 3–20.

Christiansen, C. (2007). Adolf Meyer revisited: Connections between lifestyles, resilience, and illness. *Journal of Occupational Science, 14*(2), 63–76. https://doi.org/10.1080/14427591.2007.9686586

Christiansen, C. (2021). Romanticism and transcendentalism: Ideas that made occupational therapy possible and holistic practice necessary In S. Taff (Ed.), *Philosophy and Occupational Therapy* (pp. 63–74). Slack.

Christiansen, C., & Haertl, K. (2018). A contextual history of occupational therapy. In B. S. G. Gillen (Ed.), *Willard and Spackman's Occupational Therapy* (pp. 11–41). Lippincott Williams & Wilkins.

Clark, F. A., Parham, D., Carlson, M. E., Frank, G., Jackson, J., Pierce, D., ... & Zemke, R. (1991). Occupational science: Academic innovation in the service of occupational therapy's future. *The American Journal of Occupational Therapy*, 45(4), 300–310.

Clark, F. (2006). One person's thoughts on the future of occupational science. *Journal of Occupational Science, 13*(2–3), 167–179.

Classen, S. (2018). Growth and advances of OTJR. *OTJR: Occupation, Participation and Health*, 38(1), 3–5.

Cruz, D. M. C., Taff, S., & Davis, J. (2023). Occupational engagement: Some assumptions to inform occupational therapy. *Cadernos Brasileiros de Terapia Ocupacional, 31*, e3385. https://doi.org/10.1590/2526-8910.ctoAR259233852

Dunton, W. R., Jr. (1919). *Reconstruction therapy*. WB Saunders Company.

Fisher, A. G. (2014). Occupation-centred, occupation-based, occupation-focused: Same, same or different? *Scandinavian Journal of Occupational Therapy, 21*(Suppl 1), 96–107. https://doi.org/10.3109/11038128.2014.952912

Geiger, R. L. (2014). *The history of American higher education*. Princeton University Press.

Gutman, S. A., Mortera, M. H., Hinojosa, J., & Kramer, P. (2007). Revision of the occupational therapy practice framework. *The American Journal of Occupational Therapy, 61*(1), 119.

Hammell, K. W. (2004). Dimensions of meaning in the occupations of daily life. *Canadian Journal of Occupational Therapy, 71*(5), 296–305.

Hammell, K. W. (2009). Sacred texts: A sceptical exploration of the assumptions underpinning theories of occupation. *Canadian Journal of Occupational Therapy, 76*(1), 6–13.

Henk, A. M., & Ten Have, J. (1987). Medicine and the Cartesian image of man. *Theoretical Medicine, 8*(2), 235–246. https://doi.org/10.1007/bf00539758

Kielhofner, G., & Burke, J. P. (1980). A model of human occupation, part 1. Conceptual framework and content. *The American Journal of Occupational Therapy, 34*(9), 572–581.

Kiepek, N. C., Beagan, B., Rudman, D. L., & Phelan, S. (2019). Silences around occupations framed as unhealthy, illegal, and deviant. *Journal of Occupational Science, 26*(3), 341–353.

Kennedy, J., & Davis, J. A. (2017). Clarifying the construct of occupational engagement for occupational therapy practice. *The Occupation Therapy Journal of Research: Occupation, Participation and Health, 37*(2), 98–108. https://doi.org/10.1177/1539449216688201

Levine, R. (1987). The influence of the arts-and-crafts movement on the professional status of occupational therapy. *The American Journal of Occupational Therapy, 41*(4), 248–254. https://doi.org/10.5014/ajot.41.4.248

Luchins, A. S. (1988). The rise and decline of the American asylum movement in the 19th century. *The Journal of Psychology, 122*(5), 471–486.

Marmot, M., & Wilkinson, R. (Eds.). (2005). *Social determinants of health*. Oxford University Press.

Meyer, A. (1922). The philosophy of occupation therapy. Reprinted from the *Archives of Occupational Therapy*, Volume 1, pp. 1–10, 1922. *The American Journal of Occupational Therapy: Official Publication of the American Occupational Therapy Association, 31*(10), 639–642.

Nelson, D. L. (1988). Occupation: Form and performance. *The American Journal of Occupational Therapy: Official Publication of the American Occupational Therapy Association, 42*(10), 633–641. https://doi.org/10.5014/ajot.42.10.633

Parry, M. (2010). From a patient's perspective: Clifford Whittingham Beers' work to reform mental health services. *American Journal of Public Health, 100*(12), 2356–2357.

Reed, K. L. (2005). Dr. Hall and the work cure. *Occupational Therapy in Health Care, 19*(3), 33–50. https://doi.org/10.1080/J003v19n03_04

Reilly, M. (1963). The Eleanor Clarke Slagle: Occupational therapy can be one of the great ideas of 20th century medicine. *Canadian Journal of Occupational Therapy, 30*(1), 5–19.

Richards, K. C., Enderlin, C. A., Beck, C., McSweeney, J. C., Jones, T. C., & Roberson, P. K. (2007). Tailored biobehavioral interventions: A literature review and synthesis. *Research and Theory for Nursing Practice, 21*(4), 271–285.

Rutkow, I. (2012). *Seeking the cure: A history of medicine in America.* Scribner.

Sackett, D. L., Rosenberg, W. M., Gray, J. M., Haynes, R. B., & Richardson, W. S. (1996). Evidence-based medicine: What it is and what it isn't. *British Medical Journal, 312*(7023), 71.

Society for the Study of Occupation (2019). *Position statement on the relationships between occupational science and occupational therapy.* https://ssou.memberclicks .net/assets/docs/2020-01-16_SSO-USA_Position_Statement.pdf

Tickle-Degnen, L. (2000). Teaching evidence-based practice. *The American Journal of Occupational Therapy, 54*(5), 559–560.

Townsend, E., & Wilcock, A. (2004). Occupational justice. In C. H. Christiansen & E. Townsend (Eds.), *Introduction to occupation: The art and science of living* (pp. 243–273), Prentice-Hall.

Twinley, R., Ed. (2021). *Illuminating the dark side of occupation. International perspectives from occupational therapy and occupational science.* Routledge.

Van Tubergen, A., & Van Der Linden, S. (2002). A brief history of spa therapy. *Annals of the Rheumatic Diseases, 61*(3), 273–275. https://doi.org/10.1136/ard.61.3.273

Vikat, A., & Boko, D. (2013). Chapter 1: Introduction (pp. 6–10). In *Task Force for Time Use Surveys Monograph: Guidelines for harmonizing time use surveys.* Developed by the Task Force for Time Use Surveys at the *United Nations Economic Commission for Europe, Conference of European Statisticians,* Third Meeting, Luxemburg,5–6 February, 2013.

West, W. L. (1981). The need, the response: "Occupational Therapy Journal of Research": Message from the President. *American Journal of Occupational Therapy, 35*(1), 44. https://doi.org/10.5014/ajot.35.1.44

White, R. W. (1959). Motivation reconsidered: The concept of competence. *Psychological Review, 66*(5), 297.

White, R. W. (1971). The urge towards competence. *American Journal of Occupational Therapy, 25,* 271–274.

Wilcock, A. A. (2006). *An occupational perspective of health.* Slack Incorporated.

World Federation of Occupational Therapy. (2022). *Definitions of Occupational Therapy from Member Organizations.* https://wfot.org/resources/definitions-of-occupational -therapy-from-member-organisations

World Federation of Occupational Therapy (2022). About occupational therapy: Definition of occupation. https://wfot.org/about/about-occupational-therapy

Yerxa, E. J. (1967). Authentic occupational therapy, 1966 Eleanor Clarke Slagle lecture. *American Journal of Occupational Therapy, 21*(1), 1–9.

Yerxa, E. J. (1980). Occupational therapy's role in creating a future climate of caring. *American Journal of Occupational Therapy, 34*(8), 529–534.

Yerxa, E. J., Clark, F., Frank, G., Jackson, J., Parham, D., Pierce, D., ... & Zemke, R. (1989). Occupational science: The foundation for new models of practice. *Occupational Therapy in Health Care,* 6(4), 1–17. https://doi.org/10.1080/J003v06n04_04

Chapter 2

How Everyday Occupations Influence Health and Well-being

Introduction

Occupational therapy was founded on a firm belief that occupation was not only curative and restorative, but essential for health and well-being (Andersen & Reed, 2017). Yet, in its early years, the scientific evidence for these benefits was mostly anecdotal and based on tradition, observation, and experience. A century later, considerable research across multiple disciplines has provided empirical validation for the benefits of human occupation, providing acknowledgment for its pivotal influence on the health of individuals and populations.

In this book, the World Health Organization (WHO) definition of health, written in its founding documents, underlies all uses of the term well-being:

> Health is a state of complete physical, mental, and social well-being and not merely the absence of disease or infirmity. The enjoyment of the highest attainable standard of health is one of the fundamental rights of every human being without distinction of race, religion, political belief, economic or social condition.
>
> (WHO, 1948, p. 22).

Two aspects of this definition deserve special attention. First, health and well-being are seen as fundamental rights, entitled to all. Second, inclusion of the term "social well-being" explicitly extends the scope of health (and thus health-related services) beyond the traditional physical and mental domains to include those living circumstances that influence people's health. This includes such concerns as where people live, what they do, how they meet economic requirements for daily living, and their access to food, education, and vital health-related services. These are social factors that are collectively called "**social determinants of health**" (SDOH). Importantly, these social determinants involve everyday human occupations.

Inclusion of the term "social well-being" in the definition also deserves attention. Does social well-being mean the health of populations, life satisfaction,

DOI: 10.4324/9781003242185-2

quality of life, or all of these? Since its introduction, many scholars have criticized the inadequacies and ambiguities of the WHO definition of health, seeing it as too broad, idealistic, and difficult to measure. Perhaps no observer has summarized the widespread criticism of the WHO definition with more humor and wit than Daniel Callahan (1973, p. 77), a respected ethicist, who once wrote: "one of the grandest games is that version of 'king of the hill' where the objective is to upset the World Health Organization (WHO) definition of health." Callahan (1973) would have preferred that the definition be less idealistic, more practical, and more focused on biological health. Yet, after 75 years of criticism about its imperfections by Callahan and others, the WHO definition has not been revised.

Instead, the idealism and ambiguity in its terminology have broadened thinking about the importance of social and economic conditions that improve quality of life and promote the health of communities and populations. Over time, this broader view of health has resulted in the widespread inclusion of the term "well-being" as a purpose of occupational therapy, especially as the profession has become less influenced by medicine (AOTA, 2015). Occupational science has also helped broaden this view.

What Is Well-Being?

Aldrich (2011) noted that use of the term "well-being" in the literature of occupational science (OS) and occupational therapy (OT) has been inconsistent and devoid of an established, agreed-upon meaning. Her analysis of the literature concluded that if well-being is to become a useful standard for studying the health-related benefits of occupation, researchers will need to be more precise, complete, and consistent in their uses of the term.

For example, the five item *WHO-5 Well-being Index* (Topp et al., 2015), supported by the World Health Organization and developed over many years, has been translated into many languages. Yet even this index lacks a precise definition of well-being and measures feelings that seem to describe a person's current overall mood, energy, and perceived stress.

Simons and Baldwin (2021), provided a critical review of well-being definitions and proposed a universal definition of well-being: "Well-being is a state of positive feelings and meeting full potential in the world. It can be measured subjectively and objectively, using a salutogenic approach." A **salutogenic** approach is one that contributes to health and resilience to disease. The Simons and Baldwin definition is worth noting because it differentiates well-being from definitions of health and wellness and focuses on positive states (such as life satisfaction) rather than defining well-being as the absence of disease.

Diener (Diener, Lucas & Oishi, 2018, p. 1), a leading psychological researcher who focused on measuring subjective well-being (SWB), defined the concept as a positive state that described "the extent to which a person believes or feels that his or her life is going well." Yet in a review of SWB research, he concluded that much more research is needed to determine the extent to which general measures of satisfaction relate to situational factors *and* health outcomes (Diener 2013). One of the situational factors that would be of interest to occupational scientists would include participation in purposeful occupations. Klug and Maier (2015) have shown that SWB is related to goal progress in many studies.

Seligman (2011), another scientist studying well-being, developed a framework known by the acronym PERMA. The **PERMA model** lists five factors as necessary for well-being. Research on this model has found promising evidence of its validity (Wagner et al., 2020). Key components of PERMA (an acronym) include:

1) having *positive* emotions,
2) being *engaged* in an activity,
3) having good *relationships* with other people,
4) finding *meaning* in one's life, and
5) having a sense of *accomplishment* in the pursuit of one's goals.

Three characteristics of the PERMA framework stand out: First, biological health status is *not* included as a factor necessary for well-being. Seligman (2018) has identified health for possible inclusion in future versions. Second, Seligman's definition explicitly refers to *activity engagement, meaning*, and *goal accomplishment*. This directly connects it to occupational therapy definitions and concepts. Third, the definition recognizes the importance of *positive relationships with other people*, thus connecting it to the WHO definition of heath.

In summary, both well-being and health describe positive states represented by overlapping but distinct terms defined in different ways. The multifaceted nature of these concepts includes biological, psychological, and sociological factors. This supports a view that they are best understood using a **biopsychosocial model** framework, a conceptual model to be introduced in the next section.

Organizing the Literature: A Biopsychosocial Approach

The term "biopsychosocial" is often incorrectly credited to George Engel (1977), a physician who proposed the model as a suitable replacement for the existing medical model, which had been used for decades to guide medical practice based on biological knowledge. In the medical model the *absence of disease* is considered the aim of treatment. Engel's paper in the prestigious journal *Science* got the attention of the medical community (Lugg, 2022). Among others, occupational therapy scholar Ann Mosey (1974) had published a paper with a similar title and perspective over a decade prior to Engel's work. Unfortunately,

Mosey's paper was published before most occupational therapists were able to appreciate its significance.

However, Engel's paper did have impact in the medical community. He argued that research had demonstrated that health problems must be understood as much more than simply disorders in a biological system. Citing general systems theory, Engel proposed that a new holistic model that went beyond biological medicine was needed to understand health and illness. **General systems theory** is a widely accepted view that every entity in the universe is a system or part of another system; and that systems cannot be adequately understood by simply knowing their components (von Bertalanffy, 1950). Based on systems theory, Engel concluded that health could only be fully understood by viewing it in a biopsychosocial manner.

These perspectives were getting similar attention in occupational therapy at the same time. For example, Kielhofner (1978) also proposed that a full understanding of human occupation required a biopsychosocial approach based on general systems theory. He argued that the study of human occupation would reveal how people *experienced* their states of health from the standpoint of everyday living.

Around that time, Tristram Engelhardt Jr, MD, PhD, a medical philosopher, observed that "People are healthy or diseased in terms of the activities open to

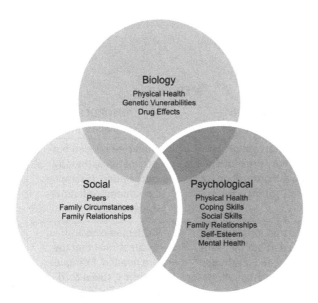

Figure 2.1 The biopsychosocial model describes three important domains of health (Seth Falco, Creative Commons license from wikimedia.org. https://tinyurl .com/ybs33caz)

them or denied them" (1977, p. 667). Engelhardt argued that people with illness were less concerned about their diagnoses than they were about how their conditions limited their engagement in valued activities. In framing health and disease in this way, Engelhardt was proposing that occupational therapy provided an important and necessary bridge between the disease-centered world of medicine and the everyday experiences and lives of individuals.

To further emphasize this point, occupational therapy scholar Joan Rogers (1982) wrote an influential paper about the sharp distinction between occupational therapy and medicine. She pointed out that in occupational therapy, disorders are properly understood as a person's inability to engage fully in the occupations they need and want to do, whereas in medicine, disorders are mostly viewed as biological problems. She observed that there are many instances where people are biologically healthy yet are unable to fulfill important life activities satisfactorily or competently and can thus benefit from occupational therapy intervention. Rogers did not suggest that medical approaches were without value; she simply noted that they were often *insufficient* to fully address the conditions that interfered with a person's engagement in the **meaningful occupations** of life. Kielhofner, Engelhardt and Rogers were all implicitly acknowledging that the biopsychosocial framework for health was better suited to occupational therapy than perspectives grounded in medicine (see Figure 2.2).

MEDICINE

		ORDER= (Health)	DISORDER= (Disease)
OCCUPATIONAL THERAPY	**ORDER=** OCCUPATIONAL PERFORMANCE	No intervention or primary prevention and health promotion for well populations.	Medicine needed but occupational therapy not needed. (Examples: pneumonia, influenza appendicitis)
	DISORDER= OCCUPATIONAL PERFORMANCE DYSFUNCTION	Occupational therapy needed but medicine unneeded. Example: housing adaptations for normal aging.	Both medicine and occupational therapy are needed. Examples: Arthritis, spinal cord injury, brain injury.

Figure 2.2 Occupational therapy and medicine define health in different ways (adapted from Rogers, 1982)

The Biopsychosocial Framework and Occupational Therapy History

The history of occupational therapy over its first century included periods of emphasis on the different domains of the biopsychosocial framework (Kielhofner, 1977). For example, the field emerged as an approach to mental illness, showing how occupation affected both psychological and social domains of health. Later, to increase its perceived legitimacy in health care, occupational therapy partnered with medicine and focused its efforts in a biologically centered manner (Andersen & Reed, 2017). During this period the field emphasized how the muscles and movements involved in completing specific tasks could be employed to improve strength or coordination; thus rehabilitating limbs or restoring the neurological patterns underlying movement. In a parallel manner, therapists working with psychiatric patients (the term used at the time) could divert a patient's obsessive behaviors, reduce anxiety, promote relaxation, and provide opportunities for supervised socialization through arts, crafts, and recreational activities. These interventions were designed to be both diversional and restorative, since therapists were taught to engage clients with activities based on the presumed underlying mental processes associated with their materials and methods (Andersen & Reed, 2017; Serrett, 1985).

Then, as occupational science emerged in the 1990s, greater emphasis was placed on community-based interventions that promoted health and prevented disease through targeted programs, often focusing on older adults (Stav et al., 2012). A multi-domain recognition of occupation-related intervention has continued into the 21st century, as occupational science and occupational therapy work together to develop a science-based understanding of occupation and health using the biopsychosocial framework.

The biopsychosocial framework is used by other disciplines, but in occupational science and occupational therapy, it is viewed through the perspective of occupation (Njelesani et al., 2014). Wilcock (1998; 2006) described this as an **occupational perspective of health**, which she defined as "a particular view of health from the perspective of humans as occupational beings" (p. 97). Wilcock's definition of occupational perspective is ideally suited as a lens for identifying how human occupation is influenced by biological, psychological, and social factors.

Established Relationships between Doing and Health

The question of how occupation (and occupational therapy) influence health in the biological, psychological, and social domains is addressed in the remainder of this chapter. The scientific literature on known relationships between occupation (or activity) and health is enormous, and several scoping reviews and metanalyses have been published in the OS and OT literature (e.g., Creek & Hughes, 2008; Gutman & Schindler, 2007). The purpose here is not to summarize or augment those reviews, but to provide examples from the research literature that demonstrate relationships between occupation and outcomes associated with each of the three domains.

While many of the studies to be referenced in this discussion are primarily focused on outcomes in a single domain, for example, how various types of regular physical exercise reduce blood pressure—a biological outcome—(Romero et al, 2017), other research illustrates how an activity can affect more than one domain. For example, mindfulness meditation can change the brain's physiological relaxation response (biological domain), yet also improve mood and emotion (psychological domain) (e.g., Zeidan et al., 2014).

Occupation and the Biological Domain

The bulleted examples below provide a glimpse into the use of occupation to prevent adverse consequences or improve function through mechanisms of action in the **biological domain**. Although these studies describe relationships between specific types of occupation and specific biological systems, one can easily imagine how similar outcomes might be obtained using other kinds of occupations.

- Regular physical occupations are associated with improved cardiovascular health, and lower hypertension (Wang et al., 2017).
- Regular challenging activity involving movement is associated with joint mobility, bone development, muscle strength, and coordination (Le Roux et al., 2022).
- Yoga and mindfulness meditation can reduce stress as measured by physiological measures of stress (allostatic load) (Pascoe et al., 2017).
- Regular active engagement in mentally stimulating occupations induces neural changes in the brain associated with maintaining cognitive function and reduced risk of dementia (Christie et al., 2017; Yates et al., 2016).

It is important to reemphasize the multi-domain benefits of certain occupational pursuits. Consider participating in a chess club or playing ultimate frisbee. These can respectively provide cognitive or physiological benefits, yet they also involve social interactions that can influence feelings of enjoyment, accomplishment, or acceptance, which involve the psychological and social domains.

Activities involving movement provide additional examples. Sustained lack of movement can result in muscle stiffness and rigidity, loss of muscle mass, skin sores, weight gain, and blood clots (Dittmer & Teasell, 1993). Similarly, sedentary behavior and immobility are associated with many chronic diseases (Dempsey et al., 2020; Le Roux et al., 2022). **Disuse syndrome** and **sensory deprivation** can also result from prolonged inactivity due to lengthy hospitalizations related to critical care or chronic illness (Fernandes et al., 2015), or from environmental conditions devoid of opportunities for sensory stimulation or social interaction (Leigh-Hunt et al., 2017). Similar consequences can result from prolonged incarceration, or conditions resulting from refugeeism, natural disasters, and wars that place individuals in sensory or socially deprived **environments** (Whiteford, 2010).

The pandemic of 2020 provided a vivid example of how social isolation and sensory deprivation can occur within health care facilities. Individuals with acute respiratory distress syndrome during the Covid-19 pandemic were often treated in intensive care units. These spaces were ideal for *biological recovery*, but seldom ideal places for *healing*. This is because they often lacked characteristics that promoted rest, facilitated supportive social interaction, or provided cognitive stimulation; all of which are necessary for healing (Verderber et al., 2021). Healing is more than physiological curing; it also involves the *experience* of enduring and moving beyond suffering and adversity. Ideal healing environments require care practices and approaches and enriched environments that consider biological, psychological, social, and spiritual needs (Firth et al., 2015).

An occupational perspective on health requires understanding the distinction between physiological recovery and healing, it also requires an appreciation that illness affects people in biological, psychological, and social ways. Occupational therapists are educated to consider the places where people live and work and to identify how those places can be changed to enhance abilities or enrich the experiences within them. There is a growing literature in health care and design about making care settings more livable and human (e.g., Bell et al., 2018). These characteristics not only relate to architectural features such as lighting, noise, and accessibility, but also pertain to the attitudes, knowledge, and skills of people (including care providers) within the environment.

Occupation and the Psychological Domain

The domain of psychological health and its reciprocal interactions with occupation is vast. As a result, beyond issues of motivation, personality, and emotion, the psychological domain includes concepts such as goal attainment, habits, competence, self-concept, identity, spirituality, and personal meaning.

The bullets below illustrate a representative sample of how occupations influence some of the psychological factors listed above as documented in the literature.

- Regular participation in Tai Chi improves mood and reduces levels of perceived stress, depression, and anxiety (Wang et al., 2010).
- Consistent daily routines and habits can improve sleep, role function, and mood. Disrupted routines are associated with depression, bipolar disorder, metabolic disorders, and insomnia (Haynes et al., 2016).

- Successful progress in attaining valued goals is associated with improved subjective well-being (Kaftan & Freund, 2018).
- Physically active lifestyles are associated with positive mood (happiness), improved self-esteem and reduced levels of depression and anxiety (Zhang & Chen, 2019).

Not represented in the examples above is an extensive literature about various psychological disorders and their occupational or lifestyle consequences. Bipolar disorder, for example, a psychological condition with fluctuating mood that includes depression as well as mania, results in a disordered lifestyle that bounces from periods of inactivity to hyperactivity. These extreme variations in activity level can interfere with interpersonal relationships, sleep, nutrition, and paid work (Gitlin & Miklowitz, 2017). Normalization of everyday lifestyle routines for people with bipolar disease (Frank et al., 2019) is recognized as a useful approach for this condition. This approach is reminiscent of early practices in occupational therapy's history.

The overlap between psychological and social factors can sometimes be confusing when one is trying to determine if a particular influence on health should be included in the psychological or social domain of the biopsychosocial framework. As a result, some of these health consequences are described as psychosocial in nature. Perhaps a useful way to deal with this ambiguity is to consider whether the psychological factor being considered is a characteristic of the individual (e.g., a behavior, an attitude, a personality trait, an emotion, or a **habit**). Such factors are usually categorized as belonging in the **psychological domain**. In contrast, influences on health status from outside the individual (such as those related to groups, communities, and cultures) typically belong in the social domain. These interfaces between the two domains demonstrate the multiple interconnections specified in general systems theory.

Occupation and the Social Domain

Occupations are inherently social. That is, they are named by the **culture**, often done for or with others (directly or indirectly), and as discussed above, their performance or engagement often relates to fulfilling social role obligations and responsibilities. Roles and responsibilities are expectations created by social groups as a way of organizing and sustaining collective living. Thus, not surprisingly, the **social domain** has many elements that have an impact on health, whether involving the health of individuals, groups, or populations (Berkman et al., 2014). These include the arrangement of homes and communities to foster safety, cooperation, proximity to food and clean water, transportation, and access to public services. Even social capital, defined as the degree of cooperation and trust within groups (Moore & Kawachi, 2017) has been shown to influence the health of communities (Xue et al., 2020). Note these same social factors apply to temporary housing conditions such as refugee camps.

Even within this brief description of groups and communities, it is easy to identify social factors that influence health and are related to daily occupations and lifestyles. Urbanization and industrialization in the United States created group living challenges related to health and safety that led to the emergence of public health as an organized discipline in 1872 (Rosen, 2015). Later, public health became distinct from medicine, leading to the evolution of federal, state, and local authorities created to promote health and prevent disease. Beginning in the 1990s, the term "**population health**" was introduced. Over time, the terms have often been used interchangeably, although there is not consensus as to whether they have distinct meanings (Roux, 2016). Both terms refer to organized efforts to improve systems of delivery and outcomes for groups.

Yet, organized efforts to address socioeconomic disparities, including those related to housing, nutrition, working conditions, access to health care, maternal health, and other social factors, often become embroiled in political debates about the social responsibilities of communities toward individual citizens (Rosen, 2015). For example, the pandemic of 2020 demonstrated that efforts to address the broad scope of social factors influencing health was quite variable and often depended on local traditions and sentiments (Schneider, 2021).

The examples shown below provide a very small glimpse into the broad range of topics pertinent to social factors as these are related to lifestyles and human occupation.

- Community-based intervention programs focusing on managing living skills for persons with dementia and their family caregivers improves daily functioning and perceived caregiving competence (Backhouse et al., 2017).
- Occupation-based, lifestyle-focused preventive health programs with older adults living in the community improves functional status, health perception, mental status, and life satisfaction (Clark et al., 1997; Jackson et al., 2009).
- Community-based programs focusing on self-management of chronic disease or leisure education improve leisure participation in older adults (Smallfield & Molitor, 2018).
- Multi-component population-based intervention programs with exercise, fall prevention education, and environmental modification to abate hazards improves quality of life and reduces the frequency and consequences of falls in community-dwelling elderly persons (Elliott & Leland, 2018).

A review of the literature in occupational therapy shows that, despite their potential, population-oriented practices for health promotion and disease prevention by occupational therapists are still in their infancy. Many professional articles in occupational therapy (e.g., Bass & Baker, 2017; Reitz & Scaffa, 2020) have called for greater attention to the social determinants of health as articulated by the World Health Organization (2008). Programs to promote healthier lifestyles in specific populations are especially needed, such as with older adults and persons with disabilities, including those with intellectual disabilities (Overwijk et al., 2021; Frank, 2015).

Wilcock (1998) inspired occupational therapists to imagine greater global participation in disease prevention and health promotion over two decades ago. She noted that social inequities affecting participation in paid work and valued activities have health consequences, and that these should be viewed as a social justice issue. This has led to emergence of the concept of occupational justice in the occupational therapy literature (Hocking, 2017). This concept will be discussed later in the book.

BOX 2.1 THE POINT IS:

- Health is influenced by many social determinants, including the social capital of communities, economic conditions, and having lifestyles that permit engagement in valued occupations.
- In addition to positive emotions and relationships, having meaning in life and being able to satisfy goals and engage in activities are also viewed as important factors in well-being, a concept distinct from health.
- The biopsychosocial framework organizes knowledge about influences on health and wellness from biological, psychological, and social domains.
- Despite abundant scientific research showing how daily occupations influence health (and vice versa), only a small portion of this knowledge is currently applied in occupational therapy practice.

References

Aldrich, R. M. (2011). A review and critique of well-being in occupational therapy and occupational science, *Scandinavian Journal of Occupational Therapy*, *18*(2), 93–100, https://doi.org/10.3109/11038121003615327

American Occupational Therapy Association (AOTA). (2015). Standards of practice for occupational therapy. *American Journal of Occupational Therapy*, *69*(Suppl. 3), 6913410057. http://dx.doi.org/10.5014/ajot.2015.696S06

Andersen, L. T., & Reed, K. L. (2017). *The history of occupational therapy: The first century*. Slack.

Backhouse, A., Ukoumunne, O. C., Richards, D. A., McCabe, R., Watkins, R., & Dickens, C. (2017). The effectiveness of community-based coordinating interventions in dementia care: A meta-analysis and subgroup analysis of intervention components. *BMC Health Services Research, 17*(1), 1–10.

Bass, J. D., & Baker, N. A. (2017). Occupational therapy and public health: Advancing research to improve population health and health equity. *OTJR: Occupation, Participation and Health, 37*(4), 175–177.

Bell, S. L., Foley, R., Houghton, F., Maddrell, A., & Williams, A. M. (2018). From therapeutic landscapes to healthy spaces, places and practices: A scoping review. *Social Science & Medicine, 196*, 123–130.

Berkman, L. F., Kawachi, I., & Glymour, M. M. (Eds.). (2014). *Social epidemiology.* Oxford University Press.

Callahan, D. (1973). The WHO definition of "health." *Hastings Center Studies*, 77–87.

Christie, G. J., Hamilton, T., Manor, B. D., Farb, N. A., Farzan, F., Sixsmith, A., Temprado, J. J., & Moreno, S. (2017). Do lifestyle activities protect against cognitive decline in aging? A review. *Frontiers in Aging Neuroscience, 9*, 381. https://doi.org/10.3389/fnagi.2017.00381

Clark, F., Azen, S. P., Zemke, R., Jackson, J., Carlson, M., Mandel, D., ... & Lipson, L. (1997). Occupational therapy for independent-living older adults: A randomized controlled trial. Journal of the American Medical Association (*JAMA*), *278*(16), 1321–1326.

Creek, J., & Hughes, A. (2008). Occupation and health: A review of selected literature. *British Journal of Occupational Therapy, 71*(11), 456–468.

Dempsey, P. C., Matthews, C. E., Dashti, S. G., Doherty, A. R., Bergouignan, A., Van Roekel, E. H., ... & Lynch, B. M. (2020). Sedentary behavior and chronic disease: Mechanisms and future directions. *Journal of Physical Activity and Health, 17*(1), 52–61.

Diener, E. (2013). The remarkable changes in the science of subjective well-being. *Perspectives on Psychological Science, 8*(6), 663–666.

Diener, E., Lucas, R. E., & Oishi, S. (2018). Advances and open questions in the science of subjective well-being. *Collabra: Psychology, 4*(1), 15. https://doi.org/10.1525/collabra.115.

Dittmer, D. K., & Teasell, R. C. F. P. (1993). Complications of immobilization and bed rest. Part 1: Musculoskeletal and cardiovascular complications. *Canadian Family Physician, 39*, 1428–1432, 1435–1437.

Elliott, S., & Leland, N. E. (2018). Occupational therapy fall prevention interventions for community-dwelling older adults: A systematic review. *The American Journal of Occupational Therapy, 72*(4), 7204190040p1-7204190040p11.

Engel G. L. (1977). The need for a new medical model: A challenge for biomedicine. *Science, 196*(4286), 129–136.

Englehardt, H. T., Jr. (1977). Defining occupational therapy: The meaning of therapy and the virtues of occupation. *American Journal of Occupational Therapy, 31*(10), 666–672.

Fernandes, T., Mendes, E., Preto, L., & Novo, A. (2015). Experience of a mobilization and active exercise program on the range of motion of bedridden patients with disuse syndrome. *Journal of Rehabilitation Medicine, 47*(8), 791–792.

Firth, K., Smith, K., Sakallaris, B. R., Bellanti, D. M., Crawford, C., & Avant, K. C. (2015). Healing, a concept analysis. *Global Advances in Health and Medicine, 4*(6), 44–50.

Frank J. C. (2015). A missing piece in the infrastructure to promote healthy aging programs: Education and work force development. *Frontiers in Public Health, 2,* 287. https://doi.org/10.3389/fpubh.2014.00287

Frank, E., Swartz, H. A., & Kupfer, D. J. (2019). Interpersonal and social rhythm therapy: Managing the chaos of bipolar disorder. *The Science of Mental Health, 48*(6), 257–268.

Gitlin, M. J., & Miklowitz, D. J. (2017). The difficult lives of individuals with bipolar disorder: A review of functional outcomes and their implications for treatment. *Journal of Affective Disorders, 209,* 147–154.

Gutman, S. A., & Schindler, V. P. (2007). The neurological basis of occupation. *Occupational Therapy International, 14*(2), 71–85.

Haynes, P. L., Gengler, D., & Kelly, M. (2016). Social rhythm therapies for mood disorders: An update. *Current Psychiatry Reports, 18,* 1–8.

Hocking, C. (2017). Occupational justice as social justice: The moral claim for inclusion. *Journal of Occupational Science, 24*(1), 29–42.

Jackson, J., Mandel, D., Blanchard, J., Carlson, M., Cherry, B., Azen, S., & Clark, F. (2009). Confronting challenges in intervention research with ethnically diverse older adults: The USC Well Elderly II trial. *Clinical Trials, 6*(1), 90–101.

Kaftan, O. J., & Freund, A. M. (2018). The way is the goal: The role of goal focus for successful goal pursuit and subjective well-being. In E. Diener, S. Oishi, & L. Tay (Eds.), *Handbook of Well-being.* DEF Publishers. Online: www.zora.uzh.ch/id/eprint /147437/#:~:text=http%3A//www.nobascholar.com/chapters/20

Kielhofner, G. (1977). Occupational therapy after 60 years: An account of changing identity and knowledge. *American Journal of Occupational Therapy, 31,* 675–689.

Kielhofner, G. (1978). General systems theory: Implications for theory and action in occupational therapy. *American Journal of Occupational Therapy, 32*(10), 637–645.

Klug, H. J., & Maier, G. W. (2015). Linking goal progress and subjective well-being: A meta-analysis. *Journal of Happiness Studies, 16,* 37–65.

Leigh-Hunt, N., Bagguley, D., Bash, K., Turner, V., Turnbull, S., Valtorta, N., & Caan, W. (2017). An overview of systematic reviews on the public health consequences of social isolation and loneliness. *Public Health, 152,* 157–171.

Le Roux, E., De Jong, N. P., Blanc, S., Simon, C., Bessesen, D. H., & Bergouignan, A. (2022). Physiology of physical inactivity, sedentary behaviours and non-exercise activity: Insights from the space bedrest model. *The Journal of Physiology, 600*(5), 1037–1051.

Lugg, W. (2022). The biopsychosocial model—History, controversy and Engel. *Australasian Psychiatry, 30*(1), 55–59.

Moore, S., & Kawachi, I. (2017). Twenty years of social capital and health research: A glossary. *Journal of Epidemiology and Community Health, 71*(5), 513–517. https:// doi.org/10.1136/jech-2016-208313

Mosey, A. C. (1974). An alternative: The biopsychosocial model. *American Journal of Occupational Therapy, 28,*137–140.

Njelesani, J., Tang, A., Jonsson, H., & Polatajko, H. (2014). Articulating an occupational perspective. *Journal of Occupational Science, 21*(2), 226–235.

Overwijk, A., Hilgenkamp, T. I., van der Schans, C. P., van der Putte In, A. A., & Waninge, A. (2021). Needs of direct support professionals to support people with intellectual disabilities in leading a healthy lifestyle. *Journal of Policy and Practice in Intellectual Disabilities, 18*(4), 263–272.

Pascoe, M. C., Thompson, D. R., & Ski, C. F. (2017). Yoga, mindfulness-based stress reduction and stress-related physiological measures: A meta-analysis. *Psychoneuroendocrinology, 86,* 152–168.

Reitz, S. M., & Scaffa, M. E. (2020). Occupational therapy in the promotion of health and well-being. *American Journal of Occupational Therapy, 74*(3), 1–14.

Rogers, J. C. (1982). Order and disorder in medicine and occupational therapy. *The American Journal of Occupational Therapy, 36*(1), 29–35.

Romero, S. A., Minson, C. T., & Halliwill, J. R. (2017). The cardiovascular system after exercise. *Journal of Applied Physiology, 122*(4), 925–932.

Rosen, G. (2015). *A history of public health.* Johns Hopkins University Press.

Roux, A. V. D. (2016). On the distinction—Or lack of distinction—between population health and public health. *American Journal of Public Health, 106*(4), 619–620.

Schneider, M. J. (2021). *Introduction to public health.* Jones & Bartlett Learning.

Seligman, M. (2011). *Flourish.* Simon & Schuster.

Seligman, M. (2018). PERMA and the building blocks of well-being. *The Journal of Positive Psychology, 13*(4), 333–335.

Serrett, K. D. (1985). *History of occupational therapy in mental health.* Haworth Press.

Simons, G., & Baldwin, D. S. (2021). A critical review of the definition of "wellbeing" for doctors and their patients in a post Covid-19 era. *International Journal of Social Psychiatry, 67*(8), 984 –991.

Smallfield, S., & Molitor, W. L. (2018). Occupational therapy interventions supporting social participation and leisure engagement for community-dwelling older adults: A systematic review. *The American Journal of Occupational Therapy, 72*(4), 7204190020p1-7204190020p8.

Stav, W. B., Hallenen, T., Lane, J., & Arbesman, M. (2012). Systematic review of occupational engagement and health outcomes among community-dwelling older adults. *The American Journal of Occupational Therapy, 66*(3), 301–310.

Topp, C. W., Østergaard, S. D., Søndergaard, S., & Bech, P. (2015). The WHO-5 Well-Being Index: A systematic review of the literature. *Psychotherapy and Psychosomatics, 84*(3), 167–176. https://doi.org/10.1159/000376585

Verderber, S., Gray, S., Suresh-Kumar, S., Kercz, D., & Parshuram, C. (2021). Intensive care unit built environments: A comprehensive literature review (2005–2020). *HERD: Health Environments Research & Design Journal, 14*(4), 368–415.

Von Bertalanffy, L. (1950). An outline of general system theory. *British Journal for the Philosophy of Science, 1,* 134–165.

Wagner, L., Gander, F., Proyer, R. T., & Ruch, W. (2020). Character strengths and PERMA: Investigating the relationships of character strengths with a multidomainal framework of well-being. *Applied Research in Quality of Life, 15*(2), 307–328.

Wang, C., Bannuru, R., Ramel, J., Kupelnick, B., Scott, T., & Schmid, C. H. (2010). Tai Chi on psychological well-being: Systematic review and meta-analysis. *BMC Complementary and Alternative Medicine, 10*(1), 1–16.

Wang, L., Ai, D., Zhang, N. (2017). Exercise benefits coronary heart disease. In J. Xiao (Ed.), *Exercise for cardiovascular disease prevention and treatment: Advances in experimental medicine and biology*, vol. 1000. Springer. https://doi.org/10.1007/978 -981-10-4304-8_1

Whiteford, G. (2010). When people cannot participate: Occupational deprivation. In C. Christiansen & E. Townsend (Eds.), *Introduction to occupation: The art and science of living* (pp. 221–242). Prentice Hall/Pearson.

Wilcock, A. A. (1998). *An occupational perspective of health*. Slack.

Wilcock, A. A. (2006). *An occupational perspective of health*. Slack.

World Health Organization. (1948). *World Health Organization constitution. Basic documents, 1*, 22. World Health Organization.

World Health Organization. (2008). *Social determinants of health* (No, SEA-HE-190). WHO Regional Office for South-East Asia. World Health Organization.

Xue, X., Reed, W. R., & Menclova, A. (2020). Social capital and health: A meta-analysis. *Journal of Health Economics, 72*, 102317. https://doi.org/10.1016/j.jhealeco.2020 .102317

Yates, L. A., Ziser, S., Spector, A., & Orrell, M. (2016). Cognitive leisure activities and future risk of cognitive impairment and dementia: Systematic review and meta-analysis. *International Psychogeriatrics, 28*(11), 1791–1806.

Zeidan, F., Martucci, K. T., Kraft, R. A., McHaffie, J. G., & Coghill, R. C. (2014). Neural correlates of mindfulness meditation-related anxiety relief. *Social Cognitive and Affective Neuroscience, 9*(6), 751–759.

Zhang, Z., & Chen, W. (2019). A systematic review of the relationship between physical activity and happiness. *Journal of Happiness Studies, 20*, 1305–1322.

Chapter 3

Occupation, Identity, and Meaning

Introduction

Despite the vast number of people on earth, each person is both unique and like others in various ways. For over a century, psychologists and social scientists have been intrigued with understanding these similarities and differences as they are reflected in human behavior. Naturally, since everyday behaviors involve occupations, occupational therapists and occupational scientists are similarly interested in these phenomena, leading to questions like the following:

> Why do some people choose highly social activities for their leisure pursuits, while others prefer to be alone in nature? What are the personal characteristics that explain success in certain types of paid work? What characteristics make the same activity enjoyable to some and stressful to others? What types of activities help explain why some retired people are happier than others?

Social scientists recognize that individual characteristics, environmental characteristics, and the nature of the activities being pursued are relevant factors in addressing these questions. In this chapter the focus will be on the person-related and activity (or occupation-related) aspects of this explanation. Over lifetimes, activity choices are central to the experiences people assemble into the personal stories that give them meaning. Personal meaning refers to an individual's thoughts and feelings about the core significance and purpose of their existence. These feelings can have favorable or unfavorable implications for their life satisfaction, health, and well-being. Consider the story in Box 3.1 about Jeremy, a combat veteran.

DOI: 10.4324/9781003242185-3

BOX 3.1 JEREMY: A COMBAT VETERAN WITH PTSD

Jeremy was a popular high school athlete who enjoyed hunting and fishing. He was intelligent and an above average student academically. After high school graduation, Jeremy decided to enlist in the Marines, hoping to qualify for an elite special forces unit. He reasoned that this would give him an opportunity to learn leadership skills, keep fit, work outdoors, meet new friends in interesting places, and find a career.

Jeremy qualified for training with an elite unit and was soon assigned to Afghanistan. He loved the sense of pride and purpose associated with his work and was soon promoted. Unfortunately, during his second tour of duty, a member of his squad was killed by a landmine, and shrapnel from the explosion severely injured Jeremy's left eye, which trauma surgeons were unable to save. This disqualified Jeremy for continued duty in the special forces.

After his discharge, Jeremy returned home and struggled with PTSD and depression, unable to stay focused on any training or study programs for pursuing another career. Jeremy is now in a rehab and substance use recovery program, having become addicted to opioid pain killers. He is struggling to find a sense of meaning in his life.

Unfortunately, stories about combat veterans like Jeremy occur all too frequently. Yet, they raise important questions about how people respond to trauma and stressful situations. Two other wounded veterans in Jeremy's PTSD counseling group are now making satisfactory progress in community college or vocational training programs. They also had traumatic experiences from duty in the Middle East, yet were eventually able to learn successful coping skills through cognitive behavioral therapy. They found new goals for moving forward with their lives. They are now making steady progress in college or vocational training programs.

One approach toward explaining these different outcomes involves drawing from **personality theory** as it is viewed through an occupational lens. Recall that an occupational lens is one that views concepts from the standpoint of occupations or activities. Personality theory can often provide possible explanations for how individuals view opportunities, select activities, interpret experiences, and overcome trauma to make sense of their lives. Later, the chapter will discuss **narrative** and personal stories. As that discussion will reveal, there is a connection between personalities and stories, but they are distinctly different concepts.

Personality and Individual Differences

Most readers who have studied psychology will be aware that personality theories seek to explain individual differences between people and their typical behaviors. In this chapter, personality is viewed as a dynamic set of individual characteristics that influence motivations, choices, thoughts, values, and attitudes. Over its distinguished history, personality research has included many different theoretical traditions. These have included theories based on traits, as well as those focused on behaviorism, psychoanalysis, and humanism. This section will draw from research in several of these theoretical traditions, with particular attention given to how interests and traits combine to form **personality types** that have different preferences for activities.

Traits and Interests

Within one branch of personality research, traits and vocational **interests** form two related areas of attention. Both are significant because they influence choices in daily life, including the activities (occupations) people pursue for work and leisure. In addition to their influence on activity choices, traits and interests are also associated with how motivated and persistent people are in pursuing their activities (Mischel et al., 2007). A trait is a characteristic pattern of behavior, such as being creative, or outgoing. An interest is a consistent or stable preference or attraction toward a subject area, such as music, science, or engineering. A third group of personality traits relate to character. Such traits are less visible, less studied, and revealed over time. These widely valued character traits are often called virtues and have been grouped into six categories labeled *wisdom, courage, humanity, justice, moderation, and transcendence* (Peterson & Seligman, 2004). Studies have shown that these characteristics contribute to mental health and resilience (Niemiec, 2020). Because empirical research on virtues is still in its infancy and has not yet been directly studied in the occupational sciences, it is mentioned here only to note its emergence in personality research and the selected application of character strength-based interventions in education, organizational leadership, recovery, and wellness promotion programs (Ruch et al., 2020).

Despite considerable research, a clear understanding of the connection between traits and interests remains elusive (Cervone & Pervin, 2022). Evidence shows that interests and traits cluster into sets of characteristics that can be useful for describing general *personality types*, even though there can be substantial variability within each cluster. In pursuing this discussion on traits and interests as areas of explaining individual differences, it's useful to begin with a brief discussion of trait research.

Trait Research: The Big Five + HEXACO Models

Contemporary research on *traits* owes its early progress to a collaboration between psychologists Allport and Odbert (1936). They carefully listed words and definitions to identify 4,000 trait-related terms, which they then grouped according to the characteristics being described. Thirty years later, Allport (1966) was reporting the existence of 16 distinct trait clusters.

Today, after considerable research, trait theorists generally agree that five major dimensions can be used to explain differences between people. Although Donald Fiske (1949) was the first to identify these five factors, many researchers too numerous to list have confirmed them (Digman, 1990). These five major traits (called "the big five") are best described as general characteristics having ranges within which every person can be placed according to the degree to which that characteristic describes them. These general traits include *Openness, Conscientiousness, Extraversion, Agreeableness, and Neuroticism* (acronym: OCEAN) (John et al., 2008). Each of these major traits also has sub-traits that are called **facets** (see Table 3.1).

In the past decade, a possible sixth major trait dimension has been studied, labeled as *Honesty–Humility*, leading to the creation of the HEXACO six factor model (e.g., Zettler et al., 2020). Here, the "H" stands for both humility and honesty, represented by the facets of *sincerity, fairness, greed avoidance,* and *modesty*. The remaining factors in this model are *Emotionality, eXtraversion, Agreeableness, Conscientiousness,* and *Openness to experience*. Note that this model does not include Neuroticism, which is subsumed within the *emotionality* dimension. Adherents of the Big Five believe that *Honesty–Humility* is a facet or sub-dimension of Neuroticism and Agreeableness, and that the Honesty–Humility dimension has not amassed sufficient research support to justify changing the conclusions supporting the **Big Five Model**.

For example, *Conscientiousness,* which is defined as "the tendency to be careful, on time for appointments, to follow rules and to be hard working" is associated with being achievement-oriented, competent, orderly, dutiful, self-disciplined, and deliberate (Diener & Lucas, 2019, p. 282). Based on the description of Jeremy given in Box 3.1, one might predict that he would tend toward demonstrating a high level of conscientiousness because of his record

Table 3.1 The Big Five personality traits

Trait	Description
Openness	The tendency to appreciate new art, ideas, values, feelings, and behaviors.
Conscientiousness	The tendency to be careful, on-time for appointments, to follow rules, and be hardworking.
Extraversion	The tendency to be talkative, sociable, and to enjoy others; the tendency to have a dominant style.
Agreeableness	The tendency to agree and go along with others rather than to assert one's opinions and choices.
Neuroticism	The tendency to frequently experience negative emotions such as anger, worry, and sadness, as well as being interpersonally sensitive.

of achievement, his sense of duty in joining the Marine Corps, and the self-discipline that was required of him to qualify as a member of the special forces.

Research has shown that a person's trait strengths for these five characteristics are not only remarkably stable but validly predict behaviors such as generosity, curiosity, responses to stress, socialization, creativity, and punctuality. They are also associated with time use (activity choices), health, and educational status (McAdams & Pals, 2006).

Research on Interests: The Big Six Personality Types

A second line of personality research has pursued individual *interests* (Hurtado Rúa et al., 2019). People differ in their interests about the world around them. As noted earlier, an interest can be described as a preference or attraction toward a topic, object, or person. Interests change over time but have both innate and acquired characteristics. They can be influenced by many factors ranging from health status, environment, and social groups to age, gender, needs, attitudes, and values (Lent et al., 1994). Research has shown that, like traits, interests cluster into groups that correlate with specific categories of activities. Easily, the most well-known research supporting this observation is that of psychologist John Holland (1959).

Holland's research on interests as a basis for individual differences in activity preference is described in a well-known theory known as the **RIASEC model** that has had a very significant impact on guiding vocational choice (Armstrong et al., 2008). It has also been used for identifying leisure activities (Armstrong & Rounds, 2008). RIASEC is an acronym named from the six personality types or themes identified in the model: *Realistic, Investigative, Artistic, Social, Enterprising, and Conventional* (see Figure 3.1).

The RIASEC model is the scientific basis for the *Dictionary of Occupational Titles* (DOT) and its online successor, the *Occupational Information Network* (O*Net) used by the United States Department of Labor. It is likely that Jeremy, the wounded veteran whose story was referenced earlier, would be classified as a "Doer" or *Realistic* type because of his preference for physical activity and outdoor work, his active, hands-on nature, and his task-driven orientation.

Relating Personality Traits and Types

Except for the Neuroticism (Emotionality) factor, research has shown significant relationships between personality trait factors in the Big Five and Interest Types in the (**Big Six**) RIASEC model (Larson et al., 2002). It is believed that trait dimensions and Interest types are related to each other through **motivation** (Schinka et al., 1997). People differ in how their interests rather than their **personality traits** influence their behavior. Some people are motivated to strive for accomplishment while others seek personal growth. Another feature of interest types is that some people prefer interacting with people (so called "people types") while others are more interested in non-human aspects of the environment (Mount et al., 2005).

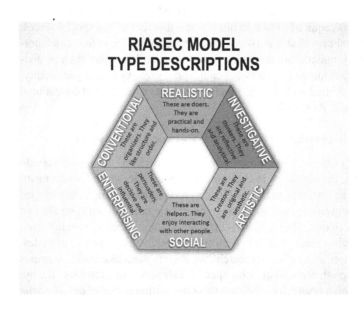

Figure 3.1 The six types of the RIASEC model (primary source: Holland, 1959)

How a person's traits, interests, and personality types influence their activity choices (both for work and leisure) is important to understanding people as occupational beings, yet very few studies have been done by researchers in occupational therapy or occupational science on this topic.

Social scientists have now recognized that a more complete view of the occupational nature of humans requires studies that consider meaningfulness, task engagement, and situational factors (Han et al., 2021). In the following section, some interesting and valuable research that has examined how people view their tasks from various perspectives is described.

Personal Projects Analysis

The concept of **personal projects** was developed by Brian Little (1983) as an approach for studying how people experience their goal-directed activities. Little defined personal projects as an "interrelated sequence of actions intended to achieve some personal goal" (Palys & Little, 1983, p. 1223). Some examples of personal projects might be "cleaning out the attic," "overcoming my fear of public speaking," "improving my relationships with co-workers," or "writing a best-selling novel."

Research has shown that individuals generally pursue 10–12 personal projects at any one time (Little et al., 2007). These studies use a novel approach known as **personal projects analysis (PPA)** (Christiansen et al., 1998). To complete a PPA, individuals list and rate their current projects according to specific dimensions or characteristics. For example, assume a person listed 12 current personal projects and the first one listed was "learning to speak Spanish". Using PPA, the individual would then rate this project (and each of their others) on a 10-point scale for each of several characteristics, such as its personal importance, its enjoyability, how meaningful it is, and several others (see Table 3.2). Rating all the characteristics or dimensions for each project currently being undertaken can require around 30 minutes or more, depending on the number of projects and the number of dimensions being rated. Any number of dimensions may be studied, but a core group of dimensions has been used across many studies (Little & Gee, 2007). The ratings for a person's individual projects are then computed and statistically analyzed.

Personal project analysis has potential for scientists in occupational therapy and occupational science because it is integrative (Christiansen et al., 1998). That is, it not only identifies *what* projects occupy people at a given point in their lives, but *how they view those projects* from a variety of perspectives. Moreover, a person's individual project ratings can be compared with the project ratings of other individuals or groups. These analyses provide important qualitative data about the unique groups of tasks pursued by individuals, but it also enables quantitative comparisons. This mixture of quantitative and qualitative data represents a mixed method research approach.

Decades of work using personal projects analysis has uncovered many important insights. An important finding is that people have "**core projects,**" or highly valued pursuits to which they are deeply committed because they are seen as essential and meaningful for their lives (Little & Grant, 2007). Research with PPA continues, and findings not only validate the approach underlying it, but they also confirm the relationships between people's projects and their levels of happiness, health, and well-being (Christiansen et al., 1999). Little has described PPA as a link between trait and interest studies of personality, and life stories, which are concerned with understanding how people connect and interpret their activities over their lives (Little et al., 1992; McGregor et al., 2006).

Table 3.2 Personal projects analysis rating dimensions*

Importance to you	Likelihood of success	Absorbing and engaging
Difficult to do	Supported by others	Adequate time to do it
Visible to others	Importance to others	Progressing satisfactorily
Controlled by you	Aligned with your values	Aligned with self-identity
Initiated by you	Expresses your Autonomy	Personal responsibility
	Creates a legacy	

* Some dimensions have been rephrased from the original for clarity, and "Creates a legacy" is a more recent addition. Not shown is an item on "Stage of completion."

Life Stories

People understand their lives as unfolding stories (Polkinghorne, 1988). In fact, developmental psychologists believe that during childhood the human brain develops a particular capacity to understand events in *story form* (Bruner, 1990). By late adolescence they grasp that they are at the center of their stories, and that this constitutes their identity. They understand that all stories have a beginning, a middle, and an end, and that stories must make sense or have **coherence** (Habermas & Bluck, 2000); they begin imagining future possibilities for their lives.

The coherence of life stories is important because each person's self-narrative creates the identity that provides them with a sense of continuity, meaning, and purpose in life (McAdams et al., 2006). In McAdams' view, a person's identity is so tied to their life story that they essentially are one and the same. People understand themselves as "stories" and to a large extent their friends and family also understand them in a storied sense.

McAdams developed standardized interviews and rating criteria to enable the collection of data on thousands of life stories (McAdams, 2008). His research has found that, typically, stories are organized according to periods (or chapters) that are defined by culturally influenced goal-related events, such as completing formal education, getting married, earning a promotion, or reaching retirement. When people think of the future or imagine "the next chapter in their lives," they make choices about the activities and directions that seem "coherent" for them based on the stories they have been living (McAdams, 2006). This illustrates the key role of goal-related activities in forming, maintaining, or enhancing one's identity (Christiansen, 1999, 2000).

Life stories have been described as an integrative level of personality. Stories incorporate traits and interests as well as goal-related activities, such as personal projects (McGregor et al., 2006)). Figure 3.2 provides a visual diagram of how these concepts relate.

Studies have shown how distinct themes reflect differences in personality types. McAdams classifies stories that describe themes of achievement or accomplishment as **agentic**, while those that emphasize social or family relationships are described as **communal** (McAdams et al., 1996). McAdams also classifies people's life stories by their plots or sequences. Some stories have *redemptive* sequences and describe their lives as having successfully overcome a difficult beginning. Such stories of commitment show how some people plan their activities with the purpose of benefitting others or serving humanity. When stories describe helping those who are younger, they are described as **generative** (McAdams & Logan, 2004).

Other types of stories may have *contamination* sequences. In these accounts, what had been a satisfactory life is disrupted by an adverse event, leading to life paths that are described by the individual as difficult and unsatisfactory (McAdams & Bowman, 2001).

McAdams' research on life stories has shown significant connections between different themes and the big five personality traits described earlier. It also

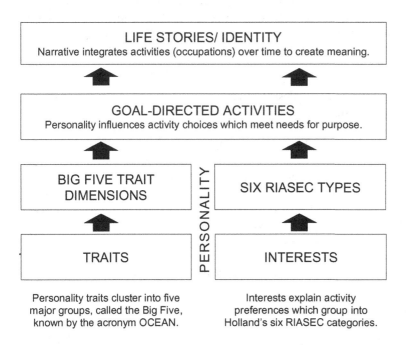

PERSONALITY
IDENTITY and MEANING
(Key concepts organized in visual form)

Figure 3.2 This diagram illustrates how key concepts in this chapter are related (source: Charles Christiansen)

demonstrates an association between story themes and measures of health and well-being (McAdams, 2011). For example, stories with *contamination* themes are often reported by people who suffer from anxiety disorders and/or depression (McAdams & Manczak, 2015); while those with *redemptive* themes are correlated with measures of psychological adaptation and life satisfaction (McAdams et al., 2001; Bauer et al., 2008).

How Stories Meet Needs for Meaning

Baumeister (Baumeister & Wilson, 1996) proposes that life stories provide an opportunity to study how four dimensions of meaning in life influence personal levels of life satisfaction. These four needs for meaning are as follows: (1) Seeing one's life as having purpose, (2) Perceiving one's life as being lived in a manner consistent with one's values and sense of justice, (3) Seeing one's life as agentic; where one's intentions can generally be achieved, and (4) Having life experiences that show approval and acceptance by others (Baumeister, 1991).

Each of these meaning needs is worthy of further elaboration, but for now, it is sufficient to mention that failing to achieve important goals, suffering through broken relationships, enduring betrayals and false accusations, or being stigmatized or rejected by others can easily be seen as experiences that could create meaning voids that make a life seem incomplete, less comprehensible, and in some cases "chaotic." Not surprisingly, people experiencing lives they feel are chaotic or incomprehensible sometimes have emotional disorders or substance use problems and can be readily found in homeless shelters and in prison populations (Greenberg & Rosenheck, 2008).

Some mental health professionals and counselors with an appreciation for the overarching significance of life stories view their roles as helping clients "reconstruct" or rewrite their life stories so that they are understood as more coherent and complete (Kerr et al., 2020). In many ways, by assisting clients to resume their important goal pursuits and participate more fully in their lives, occupational therapists are also helping people rewrite life stories (Frank, 1996). In fact, Hammell (2004) argues that a client's engagement in meaningful activity, a term used frequently in occupational therapy texts and articles, must be understood in the **context** of a client's story. Medical philosopher Tristram Engelhardt's astute observation is worth repeating here: Occupational therapists are *custodians of meaning*, in the sense that they enable people to preserve or restore meaning through intentional, life-relevant activity (Engelhardt, 1977).

Making Sense of Meaning

It is unclear when and how the word "meaning" first began appearing regularly in the occupational therapy literature. As with the term "occupation," meaning has been used to describe both process and outcome. In his often-cited paper on the philosophy of occupational therapy, Dr. Adolf Meyer (1922), emphasized the integrative value of therapy in helping the individual organize and appreciate time through opportunities to engage in occupations. Meyer believed that disordered lives (traumatic life stories) were a root cause of mental illness (Lidz, 1985). He required his medical students to construct life charts of their patients, detailing major life experiences in parallel with symptoms and episodes of ill health (Meyer, 1917). Although Meyer's paper on the philosophy of occupational therapy was given at a very early point in the evolution of psychiatry and psychology, one can imagine that his ideas were precursors to today's research on the life story as a way for the person to assign meaning to life activities and experiences and make sense of them collectively.

Yet, a century later, occupational therapy does not have a consensus definition of meaning and few writers have recently connected the concept to life stories. Often, meaningful occupation is defined as activity that is significant, motivating, and tied to purpose (Trombly, 1995). Hasselkus (2006) described meaning as an elusive, multifaceted phenomenon based on the feelings and interpretations one has of experiences.

Perhaps Eakman (2012, 2013; Eakman & Eklund, 2012; Eakman et al., 2010) has been the most productive occupational scientist studying the concepts of meaningful occupation and meaning in life. Eakman's work supports a framework in which meaningful activity meets basic needs, provides subjectively positive experiences, and contributes to a person's overall assessment of meaning in her/his life. His work is consistent with the narrative view of meaning described in this chapter. In a report describing a synthesis of studies of meaning from the *Journal of Occupational Science*, Eakman and colleagues (2018) found several common themes. These themes included *feelings* associated with the doing of the occupation, *social dimensions* associated with belonging and helping; and *selfhood dimensions*, associated with identity, autonomy, self-esteem, and other personality-related characteristics described earlier in the chapter.

Although there is no consensus about how to define meaningful occupation in occupational therapy, there are commonalities from research. These can be summarized as follows:

- Meaningful occupation is often associated with feelings of enjoyment, and satisfaction (Eakman et al., 2018).
- Meaningful occupation has a purpose that is viewed by the doer as relevant to their life, and consistent with their sense of self (Little, 2007).
- Meaningful occupation is freely chosen, challenging, and consistent with one's values (Little, 2016)).
- Meaningful occupation is related to fulfilling psychological needs and meaning in life (Eakman, 2013).

Implications for Occupational Therapy Practice

To consider how the concepts in this chapter might be applied, it is useful to return to the story of Jeremy. Recall that Jeremy's interests and personality type matched his work in the special forces. He views this period before his injury as a time when he was motivated, experiencing success, and feeling good about himself. The battlefield explosion in which his friend died altered Jeremy's vision, thinking, and his personal identity. These dramatic life changes led to depression, decreased motivation, and sleep disturbances, all of which diminished his coping abilities. Jeremy became addicted to pain medication.

Jeremy now views himself as a victim and lacks the confidence to select and pursue another career. Thematically, his life story has been *contaminated*. From a narrative standpoint, Jeremy needs to be able to "re-write" his narrative theme to one that is **redemptive**—a story of overcoming adversity.

Best practice in occupational therapy begins with an understanding of the client through the development of an occupational profile, as well as an understanding of Jeremy's work history, his interests, and preferences. An initial assessment would also gather information on Jeremy's skills and abilities for performing everyday occupations.

Occupational therapists who have expertise in the rehabilitation of persons with brain injury will complete an assessment of his ability to plan and execute tasks. Jeremy's ability to communicate as well as his mood and levels of motivation may also be assessed to consider his suitability for group cognitive behavior therapy.

If Jeremy is to re-write his story, an important first step will be for him to be taught compensatory skills to work around any deficits. For example, for memory issues, lists and reminder strategies can be employed. Strategies for improving bilateral coordination despite visual field disturbances also exist. An important feature of intervention planning is to sequence tasks so that progressive success leads to improved confidence. Digital gaming can often be adapted to foster progressive challenges.

Since each client is different, a successful approach will depend as much on the clinical reasoning and creative problem solving of the therapist as it does on the characteristics of the client. Success will always be more likely if the therapist has a better understanding of the client, since this is likely to lead to a more effective therapeutic relationship and the selection of interventions that are more meaningful to Jeremy. Jeremy's situation is complex and his progress toward improvement will be challenging.

BOX 3.2 THE POINT IS:

- Interests and traits combine to help explain personality differences and preferences for activity.
- One branch of personality research uses clusters of trait facets to explain five major personality dimensions: Openness, Conscientiousness, Extraversion, Agreeableness, and Neuroticism. These factors are called the Big Five.
- An approach to personality differences based on interest preferences involves six major types: Realistic, Investigative, Artistic, Social, Enterprising, and Conscientious. These form the basis for the categorizing work in the Dictionary of Occupational Titles.
- The study of personal narratives has shown that life stories have distinct themes that relate to life satisfaction and well-being. The coherence and continuity of stories form the basis for personal identity.
- One approach toward understanding *meaningful occupations* relates them to fulfilling psychological needs for purpose, efficacy, positive social relationships, and personal value expression.

References

Allport, G. W., & Odbert, H. S. (1936). Trait-names: A psycho-lexical study. *Psychological Monographs, 47*(1), i–171.

Allport, G. W. (1966). Traits revisited. *American Psychologist, 21*(1), 1–10.

Armstrong, P. I., Day, S. X., McVay, J. P., & Rounds, J. (2008). Holland's RIASEC model as an integrative framework for individual differences. *Journal of Counseling Psychology, 55*(1), 1–18.

Armstrong, P. I., & Rounds, J. (2008). Linking leisure interests to the RIASEC world of work map. *Journal of Career Development, 35*(1), 5–22.

Bauer, J. J., McAdams, D. P., & Pals, J. L. (2008). Narrative identity and eudaimonic well-being. *Journal of happiness studies, 9*(1), 81–104.

Baumeister, R. F. (1991). *Meanings of life.* Guilford Press.

Baumeister, R. F., & Wilson, B. (1996). Life stories and the four needs for meaning. *Psychological Inquiry, 7*(4), 322–325.

Bruner, J. S. (1990). *Acts of meaning: Four lectures on mind and culture.* Harvard University Press.

Cervone, D., & Pervin, L. A. (2022). *Personality: Theory and research.* John Wiley & Sons.

Christiansen, C. H. (1999). Defining lives: Occupation as identity: An essay on competence, coherence, and the creation of meaning. *The American Journal of Occupational Therapy, 53*(6), 547–558.

Christiansen, C. (2000). Identity, personal projects and happiness: Self construction in everyday action. *Journal of Occupational Science, 7*(3), 98–107.

Christiansen, C. H., Little, B. R., & Backman, C. (1998). Personal projects: A useful approach to the study of occupation. *The American Journal of Occupational Therapy, 52*(6), 439–446.

Christiansen, C. H., Backman, C., Little, B. R., & Nguyen, A. (1999). Occupations and well-being: A study of personal projects. *The American Journal of Occupational Therapy, 53*(1), 91–100.

Diener, E., & Lucas, R. (2019). Personality traits. In R. Biswas-Diener & E. Diener (Eds.), Noba Textbook Series: *Psychology.* DEF Publishers. nobaproject.com

Digman, J. M. (1990). Personality structure: Emergence of the five-factor model. *Annual Review of Psychology, 41*(1), 417–440.

Eakman, A. M. (2012). Measurement characteristics of the engagement in meaningful activities survey in an age-diverse sample. *The American Journal of Occupational Therapy, 66*(2), e20–e29.

Eakman, A. M. (2013). Relationships between meaningful activity, basic psychological needs, and meaning in life: Test of the meaningful activity and life meaning model. *OTJR: Occupation, Participation and Health, 33*(2), 100–109.

Eakman, A. M., & Eklund, M. (2012). The relative impact of personality traits, meaningful occupation, and occupational value on meaning in life and life satisfaction. *Journal of Occupational Science, 19*(2), 165–177.

Eakman, A. M., Carlson, M. E., & Clark, F. A. (2010). The meaningful activity participation assessment: A measure of engagement in personally valued activities. *The International Journal of Aging and Human Development, 70*(4), 299–317.

Eakman, A. M., Atler, K. E., Rumble, M., Gee, B. M., Romriell, B., & Hardy, N. (2018). A qualitative research synthesis of positive subjective experiences in occupation from the *Journal of Occupational Science* (1993–2010). *Journal of Occupational Science, 25*(3), 346–367.

EngelhardtH. T.Jr, (1977). Defining occupational therapy: The meaning of therapy and the virtues of occupation. *The American Journal of Occupational Therapy, 31*(10), 666–672.

Fiske, D. W. (1949). Consistency of the factorial structures of personality ratings from different sources. *The Journal of Abnormal and Social Psychology, 44*(3), 329.

Frank, G. (1996). Life histories in occupational therapy clinical practice. *The American Journal of Occupational Therapy, 50*(4), 251–264.

Greenberg, G. A., & Rosenheck, R. A. (2008). Jail incarceration, homelessness, and mental health: A national study. *Psychiatric Services, 59*(2), 170–177.

Habermas, T., & Bluck, S. (2000). Getting a life: The emergence of the life story in adolescence. *Psychological Bulletin, 126*(5), 748–769.

Hammell, K. W. (2004). Dimensions of meaning in the occupations of daily life. *Canadian Journal of Occupational Therapy, 71*, 296–305.

Han, S. H., Sung, M., & Suh, B. (2021). Linking meaningfulness to work outcomes through job characteristics and work engagement. *Human Resource Development International, 24*(1), 3–22.

Hasselkus, B. R. (2006). The world of everyday occupation: Real people, real lives. *The American Journal of Occupational Therapy, 60*(6), 627–640.

Holland, J. L. (1959). A theory of vocational choice. *Journal of Counseling Psychology, 6*(1), 35–45.

Hurtado Rúa, S. M., Stead, G. B., & Poklar, A. E. (2019). Five-factor personality traits and RIASEC interest types: A multivariate meta-analysis. *Journal of Career Assessment, 27*(3), 527–543.

John, O. P., Naumann, L. P., & Soto, C. J. (2008). Paradigm shift to the integrative Big Five trait taxonomy: History, measurement, and conceptual issues. In O. P. John, R. W. Robins, & L. A. Pervin (Eds.), *Handbook of Personality: Theory and Research* (pp. 114–158). The Guilford Press.

Kerr, D. J. R., Deane, F. P., & Crowe, T. P. (2020). A complexity perspective on narrative identity reconstruction in mental health recovery. *Qualitative Health Research, 30*(4), 634–649.

Larson, L. M., Rottinghaus, P. J., & Borgen, F. H. (2002). Meta-analyses of Big Six interests and Big Five personality factors. *Journal of Vocational Behavior, 61*(2), 217–239.

Lent, R. W., Brown, S. D., & Hackett, G. (1994). Toward a unifying social cognitive theory of career and academic interest, choice, and performance. *Journal of Vocational Behavior, 45*(1), 79–122.

Lidz, T. (1985). Adolf Meyer and the Development of American Psychiatry. *Occupational Therapy in Mental Health, 5*(3), 33–53. https://doi.org/10.1300/j004v05n03_02

Little, B. R. (1983). Personal projects: A rationale and method for investigation. *Environment and Behavior, 15*(3), 273–309.

Little, B. R. (2007). Prompt and circumstance: The generative contexts of personal projects analysis. In B. R. Little, K. Salmela-Aro, & S. D. Phillips (Eds), *Personal project pursuit: Goals, action, and human flourishing* (pp. 3–49). Lawrence Erlbaum.

Little, B. R. (2016). Well-doing: Personal projects and the social ecology of flourishing. *International Handbooks of Quality-of-Life*, 297–305. https://doi.org/10.1007/978-3-319-42445-3_19

Little, B. R., & Gee, T. L. (2007). The methodology of personal projects analysis: Four modules and a funnel. In B. R. Little, K. Salmela-Aro, & S. D. Phillips (Eds.), *Personal project pursuit: Goals, action, and human flourishing* (pp. 51–94). Lawrence Erlbaum.

Little, B. R., & Grant, A. M. (2007). The sustainable pursuit of personal projects, retrospect and prospect. In B. R. Little, K. Salmela-Aro, & S. D. Phillips (Eds.), *Personal project pursuit: Goals, action and human flourishing* (pp. 403–444). Lawrence Erlbaum.

Little, B. R., Lecci, L., & Watkinson, B. (1992). Personality and personal projects: Linking Big Five and PAC units of analysis. *Journal of personality*, *60*(2), 501–525.

Little, B. R., Salmela-Aro, K., & Phillips, S. D. (Eds.). (2007). *Personal project pursuit: Goals, action, and human flourishing.* Lawrence Erlbaum.

McAdams, D. P. (2006). The problem of narrative coherence. *Journal of Constructivist Psychology*, *19*(2), 109–125.

McAdams, D. P. (2008). Personal narratives and the life story In John, O, Robins, R, and Pervin L. (Eds.), *Handbook of personality: Theory and research* (pp. 241–261). Guilford Press.

McAdams, D. P. (2011). Narrative identity. In S. J. Schwartz, K. Luyckx & V. L. Vignoles (Eds.). (2011). *Handbook of identity theory and research* (pp. 99–115). Springer.

McAdams, D. P., & Bowman, P. J. (2001). Narrating life's turning points: Redemption and contamination. In D. P. McAdams, R. Josselson, & A. Lieblich (Eds.), *Turns in the road: Narrative studies of lives in transition* (pp. 3–34). American Psychological Association.

McAdams, D. P., Hoffman, B. J., Day, R., & Mansfield, E. D. (1996). Themes of agency and communion in significant autobiographical scenes. *Journal of Personality*, *64*(2), 339–377.

McAdams, D. P., Reynolds, J., Lewis, M., Patten, A. H., & Bowman, P. J. (2001). When bad things turn good and good things turn bad: Sequences of redemption and contamination in life narrative and their relation to psychosocial adaptation in midlife adults and in students. *Personality and Social Psychology Bulletin*, *27*(4), 474–485.

McAdams, D. P., & Logan, R. L. (2004). What is generativity? In E. de St. Aubin, D. P. McAdams, & T.-C. Kim (Eds.), *The generative society: Caring for future generations* (pp. 15–31). American Psychological Association.

McAdams, D. P., Josselson, R. E., & Lieblich, A. E. (2006). *Identity and story: Creating self in narrative.* American Psychological Association.

McAdams, D. P., & Manczak, E. (2015). Personality and the life story. In M. Mikulincer, P. R. Shaver, M. L. Cooper, & R. J. Larsen (Eds.), *APA handbook of personality and social psychology, Vol. 4. Personality processes and individual differences* (pp. 425–446). American Psychological Association. https://doi.org/10.1037/14343-019

McAdams, D. P., & Pals, J. L. (2006). A new Big Five: Fundamental principles for an integrative science of personality. *American Psychologist*, *61*(3), 204–217. https://doi.org/10.1037/0003-066X.61.3.204

McGregor, I., McAdams, D. P., & Little, B. R. (2006). Personal projects, life stories, and happiness: On being true to traits. *Journal of Research in Personality*, *40*(5), 551–572.

Mischel, W., Shoda, Y., & Ayduk, O. (2007). *Introduction to personality: Toward an integrative science of the person.* John Wiley & Sons.

Mount, M. K., Barrick, M. R., Scullen, S. M., & Rounds, J. (2005). Higher-order dimensions of the big five personality traits and the big six vocational interest types. *Personnel Psychology, 58*(2), 447–478. https://doi.org/10.1111/j.1744-6570.2005.00468.x

Meyer, A. (1917). Progress in teaching psychiatry. *Journal of the American Medical Association, 69*(11), 861–863.

Meyer, A. (1922). The philosophy of occupation therapy. *American Journal of Physical Medicine & Rehabilitation, 1*(1), 1–10.

Niemiec, R. M. (2020). Six functions of character strengths for thriving at times of adversity and opportunity: A theoretical perspective. *Applied Research in Quality of Life, 15*, 551–572.

Peterson, C., & Seligman, M. E. P. (2004). *Character strengths and virtues: A handbook and classification.* American Psychological Association.

Palys, T. S., & Little, B. R. (1983). Perceived life satisfaction and the organization of personal project systems. *Journal of Personality and Social Psychology, 44*(6), 1221–1230. https://doi.org/10.1037/0022-3514.44.6.1221

Polkinghorne, D. E. (1988). *Narrative knowing and the human sciences.* Suny Press.

Ruch, W., Niemiec, R. M., McGrath, R. E., Gander, F., & Proyer, R. T. (2020). Character strengths-based interventions: Open questions and ideas for future research. *The Journal of Positive Psychology, 15*(5), 680–684.

Schinka, J. A., Dye, D. A., & Curtiss, G. (1997). Correspondence between five-factor and RIASEC models of personality. *Journal of Personality Assessment, 68*(2), 355–368.

Trombly, C. A. (1995). Occupation: Purposefulness and meaningfulness as therapeutic mechanisms. *The American journal of occupational therapy, 49*(10), 960–972.

Zettler, I., Thielmann, I., Hilbig, B. E., & Moshagen, M. (2020). The nomological net of the HEXACO model of personality: A large-scale meta-analytic investigation. *Perspectives on Psychological Science, 15*(3), 723–760.

Chapter 4

How Time and Place Influence What People Do

Introduction

Time and activity can be imagined as two sides of a rolling coin. To extend the metaphor further, a coin must roll on something, and that places it in a location. Theories of occupation (and occupational therapy) agree that three essential dimensions of doing include the activity or occupation itself, the person (or people) doing it, and the place and context (or environment) in which it is done. Seldom is it specifically mentioned that doing occupations consumes time or that many occupations are done at designated times and in designated places. Additionally, the allocation of time to an activity, or the frequency with which it is done, can be an indicator of its necessity or importance. These features of everyday existence: Activity, time, and place, are usually taken for granted. Yet, they constitute important elements for fully understanding occupation and the practice of occupational therapy.

The connections between time and occupation are not new to occupational therapy. Kielhofner (1977) used the term **temporal adaptation** to describe a range of therapeutic considerations related to time and occupation, including how time is allocated across major areas of daily activity, how work and rest are balanced, how cultural expectations are met, and how time is allocated to personal meaningful pursuits across the lifetime. More recently, scholars have proposed the idea of *synchronization* (Pemberton & Cox, 2015), conceptualized as attention given to temporal rhythm and time allocation to achieve optimal alignment with physiological systems enabling activity.

The relationships between time and human occupation are of interest to scientists in other disciplines as well. Consider **time use research**. A great deal is known about how people spend time during a typical day, and this understanding comes from international time use studies. Time use research has a long history that dates to observations of peasant farm work in Russia in the late 19th century (Bauman et al., 2019). Today it is used by governments as a measure of national economic productivity, social capital, and health-related behaviors. Time use scientists have collaborated internationally to standardize

DOI: 10.4324/9781003242185-4

surveys that are used in data collection so that data can be compared globally (e.g., Gershuny, 2011).

One notable finding from multinational time use surveys is the similarity of time use patterns across nations for typical activities during a 24-hour round of daily activity. More sophisticated data collection and analysis methods are enabling scientists to analyze time use data to gather insights pertinent to well-being, such as trends in paid work hours, and time spent sleeping, or in leisure behaviors (Cornwell et al., 2019; see Figure 4.1).

Time use surveys rely on time diaries, which require respondents to recall specific amounts of time spent in various activities during the preceding 24-hour period. The validity of such diaries has been established using wearable cameras and accelerometers (Gershuny et al., 2020). The periodic collection of such data can be used to compare the time use of different age groups as well as to identify variations by gender and other demographic variables. Studies reveal gender disparities in time spent working, especially in the home, with women bearing a greater burden of household maintenance and childrearing, often through multitasking. There is emerging evidence that these disparities have health consequences (Offer & Schneider, 2011).

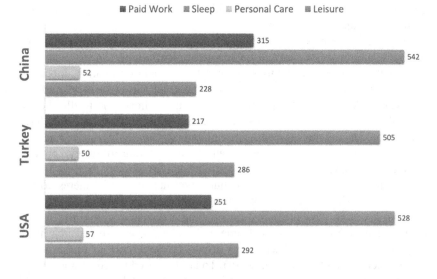

Time Use Comparisons for Selected Countries

■ Paid Work   ■ Sleep   ▨ Personal Care   ■ Leisure

China
315
542
52
228

Turkey
217
505
50
286

USA
251
528
57
292

Figure 4.1 Comparison of time use in selected countries measured in hours per week. (Charles Christiansen, data compiled from OECD online database, 2023)

Time use data have also been analyzed for insights into the relative balance of work and non-work activities (Yokying et al., 2016). Economists and sociologists have long been interested in the concept of work–life balance, and the overall concept of occupational balance is familiar to occupational therapists, having originated with **Adolf Meyer** (1922). The central idea is that well-being requires a healthy distribution of time spent in different categories of time use. The recent literature in occupational science has devoted increasing attention to the notion of *occupational balance*, but no consensus definition or conclusive evidence has emerged. There are many ways to approach the concept of balance, ranging from time allocation to needs fulfillment (Backman, 2010; Christiansen, 1996; Christiansen & Matuska, 2006; Eakman, 2016; Wagman et al., 2015). Wagman and Håkansson (2019) have noted that studies of balance are typically undertaken from an individual rather than an interpersonal perspective, arguing that research might benefit from the inclusion of broadened social perspectives.

Beyond the concept of balance, time-use research is highly germane to occupational science because it provides an objective way to identify how people *use* time. Hunt and McKay (2015) completed a scoping review of time use research by scientists in occupational therapy and occupational science between 1990 and 2014 and found 61 studies, the majority of which focused on the time use of subpopulations with different health conditions or how the time use of general populations related to health and well-being.

Time use studies have also been used to study the patterns or regularity of daily activities. Evidence suggests that regular patterns of activity are typical across individuals and even cultures. Currently, this regularity is deemed to be the result of habitual routines, biological rhythms, and societal influences, such as work scheduling or economic factors (Vagni & Cornwell, 2018).

Automaticity, Habits, and Routines

It is widely agreed that people are creatures of habit, and a new measurement scale with that name has been developed by researchers interested in habitual tendencies (Ersche et al., 2017). People tend to repeat tasks and tendencies without much thought. This forms a pattern of daily occupation that is predictable, and this consistency has both positive and negative consequences. Current theory proposes that **routine** intentional tasks are carried out by a combination of active intentional control and "automatic" subconscious behavior, with the proportions of each varying based upon the circumstances. The psychological term for the phenomenon of behaviors routinely occurring without much conscious thought is **automaticity**.

There are several features of this automatic behavior, including awareness, intention, efficiency, and control (Bargh, 1994). While a behavior can be automatic without all the features being present, automatic behaviors most often occur without much conscious awareness, sometimes creating risks. Examples

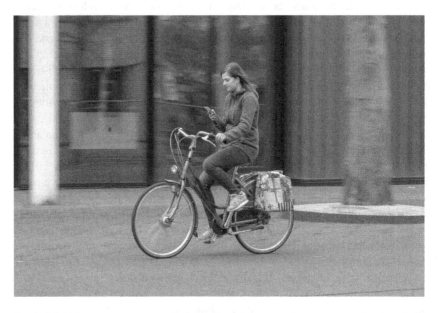

Figure 4.2 Habits are automatic behaviors—sometimes they create risks (image by Itsajoop via iStock, used under license)

include riding a bike, or even driving, which occur routinely without thinking too much about what actions are required as they occur.

Most people can recall instances when they realize that they have done something without their awareness or intention. This automatic or subconscious influence on behavior is thought to have evolved in the nervous system to help humans conserve attention and energy for more pressing needs. Social behaviors are also influenced by habit, driven by the need for social approval and other psychological factors that can influence social interaction without conscious awareness. Sometimes, reactions occur without a person being able to explain what influenced them (Bargh & Chartrand, 1999).

Because of the distinctions between the initiation of an activity and its performance, it is possible for people to consciously begin an activity that is then executed in a habitual way. Other times, people may habitually begin and then consciously complete specific tasks, such as getting dressed on a day when a special event is occurring.

Although much of routine daily behavior is automatic, typical behaviors can be disrupted depending on the situation at hand. Changes in circumstance, such as new environments and unfamiliar tasks, or even new co-workers, can have a disruptive effect on automaticity. In these cases, typically predictable behaviors become less predictable.

Health-related habits, such as oral hygiene, or regular aerobic activities, can have positive consequences. Yet, one can also develop unhealthy habits such as subconsciously eating snacks, vaping, or consuming an alcoholic beverage after psychologically stressful situations (Graybiel & Smith, 2014). Gardner (2015) suggested that complex automatic behaviors that are unhealthy can be overcome with conscious effort.

Noting the longstanding history of the concept of habit in occupational therapy, Fritz and Cutchin (2016) and Yerxa (2002) have suggested that occupational therapy practitioners are well qualified to apply knowledge about habits in planning interventions to establish healthful behaviors and routines. A useful example is a project to help well older adults remain in the community through targeted lifestyle intervention (Pyatak et al., 2022).

The Perception of Time

Although research on the individual perception of time originated over a century ago, science has made little progress in fully understanding the specific processes that help explain individual differences in time perception. Research focused on identifying specific neurological pathways shows limited success. The only consensus seems to be that this area of study is extremely complex. One approach that deserves more attention concerns situational factors that influence subjective experiences of time. Csikszentmihalyi (1990) popularized the idea of flow, or the concept that engaging activities have a timeless quality. Considerable evidence supports a connection between emotions and time perception, as for example, evidence corroborating the relationship between depression and slower temporality (e.g., Thönes, & Oberfeld, 2015). In research examining the experience of time (temporality) and its relationship to everyday activities, Larson and von Eye (2010) found that, for habitual activities, time was perceived as passing the same as clock time. More complex, novel, and skill-requiring activities or activity patterns were related to faster perceptions of time. These findings have implications for intervention planning in occupational therapy (Larson & von Eye, 2010).

Biological Rhythms

Although habits are governed by the nervous system, other regular patterns of behavior are influenced by **biological rhythms**. **Chronobiology**, the study of biological rhythms, has identified many natural cycles in the human body that have physical, mental, and behavioral effects (e.g., Zuurbier et al., 2015).

Basic Rest–Activity Cycle

The primary shorter duration (ultradian) cycle is known as the basic rest–activity cycle (BRAC). This internal arousal cycle has a duration of around 90–100 minutes and occurs both during sleep and wakefulness (Kleitman, 1982). During sleep, the BRAC has also been termed the REM (or rapid eye movement) cycle. Recent evidence has shown that the BRAC is associated with small changes in body and brain temperature that may be evolutionary in origin, designed to help the organism remain alert to changes in the physical environment (Blessing, 2018). This understanding has prompted speculation that productivity may be enhanced by taking regular breaks from mental exertion that correspond to this arousal cycle, but this has not been documented in well-controlled published studies.

Circadian Sleep–Wake Cycle

The longer duration circadian sleep–wake cycle is known to be influenced by exposure to daylight and darkness, as well as physiological processes (Aschoff & Wever, 1981). Circadian sleep–wake cycles affect a broad range of living things and are thought to have evolved to adapt organisms to the rotation of the earth and the resulting periods of night and day. These cycles coordinate internal organ systems and influence the timing of behaviors, for example, by helping bees optimize their pollination activities (Kuhlman et al., 2018).

In humans, the sleep–wake cycle recurs in a daily pattern and is regulated by hormones, primarily melatonin, operating through the hypothalamus. This internally regulated circadian cycle is synchronized by physiological pacemakers and entrained to the external environment through zeitgebers (timekeepers) that primarily react to light and temperature.

When people undertake transmeridian (multiple time zone) travel, the circadian sleep rest cycle becomes disentrained, or **desynchronized** with the environment (Arendt, 2012). The resulting condition, called Jet Lag Syndrome (desynchronosis), can result in sleep disturbance, fatigue, malaise, and gastrointestinal upset. These consequences can be prevented or remedied by careful exposure to full spectrum light and other measures.

In situations where internal clocks are not synchronized with lifestyles, daily routines are affected, and the condition is called **social jetlag** (Grandin et al., 2006). This can occur with shift work or deprived exposure to natural daylight—which may occur during incarceration or by living in polar regions where daylight is restricted. Regular human activities such as dog walks, mealtimes, or interactions with other people serve as zeitgebers for setting internal clocks (Mistlberger & Skene, 2004; 2005; see Figure 4.3).

Many physiological processes are affected by the sleep–wake cycle, including oxidative stress, immune function, heart rate, and metabolic processes, and as a result the circadian system significantly influences health (Beauvalet et al., 2017; Roenneberg et al., 2022). Many diseases show chronobiological features, and therapeutics, including surgical procedures, radiation therapy, and medications, can have greater effectiveness at certain times during the circadian cycles

INFLUENCES ON CIRCADIAN REGULATION

These normal regulating processes may be affected by illness, long distance travel, shift work, changes in the physical environment, or social disruptions that alter regular routines, such as unexpected guests, traumatic events.

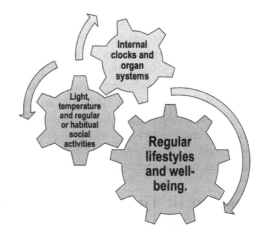

Figure 4.3 Circadian rhythms can be disrupted by biological, psychological, and social factors (Charles Christiansen, personal lecture notes)

of patients (Zaki et al., 2019). There is a growing literature in this specialized area of medicine called *chronotherapeutics.*

Each person's rhythms are unique, and research has shown that segments of the population have cycles that correspond with **morningness** or **eveningness chronotypes** (Adan et al., 2012). Not surprisingly, research has shown that chronotypes, which can be determined from questionnaires, have implications for daily routines, task performance, and susceptibility to certain conditions such as metabolic and mood disorders (Roenneberg et al., 2019).

The disruptive emotional effects of social jet lag have been described in social zeitgeber theory (Ehlers et al., 1988). Certain mental health conditions, such as bipolar disorder, have been shown to be especially susceptible to disruptions in normal patterns of daily life and dysregulation of the sleep–wake cycle. This has led to the development over the past 30 years of an instrument called the **Social Rhythm Metric** (Monk et al., 1991), which measures these disruptions for patients with bipolar illness. A behavioral approach to therapy was developed to normalize those rhythms and improve management of the disease (Frank et al., 2022). The concept of the therapeutic benefit of normalizing routines dates to the earliest days of occupational therapy, in a process called "habit training" (Slagle, 1922). Psychiatrist Adolf Meyer observed that regular routines were beneficial to the recovery of his mental patients (Meyer, 1922).

Today, therapeutic efforts to normalize circadian rhythms are often called re-entrainment or jetlag therapy. Approaches include a variety of strategies ranging from structured groups using cognitive behavioral therapy to light therapy, and medications. These therapies are often targeted at individuals with bipolar disorder but can also be beneficial for shift workers, airline employees, and others who suffer from insomnia resulting from circadian dysregulation (Fritz & Cutchin, 2016). Practitioners in occupational therapy are now providing interventions for sleep disturbance (e.g., Ho & Siu, 2018; Leland et al., 2014).

During the data gathering "occupational profile" phase of client assessment, occupational therapists should ideally screen for chronotype as well as lifestyle details that might suggest the possibility of social jet lag. This would include questions about sleep habits and quality, recent long-distance travel, or exposure to daylight in regular routines. Therapists should consider whether to schedule interventions at a time consistent with the client's chronotype.

Section II: The Concept of Place

The word **place** has many meanings, because the idea of place is "socially constructed," and given various meanings by different people, often as the result of experiences. Places can have both collective and individual meanings. For example, a park might commemorate an historical event known to a culture; but for a couple who got engaged there, its meaning is quite different.

Places have many dimensions, as reflected in the various terms used to describe them. Some terms, such as region or neighborhood, may be used to describe the general features of places. However, words such as home, community, and nation can evoke more emotional meanings. Universities, shopping centers, stadiums, parks, fairgrounds, kitchens, and bedrooms carry shared meanings that are directly tied to the occupations that occur within them.

Places as Archetypes

Hamilton (2010) noted that the first experienced environment for all humans is the uterus, and the experiences of the physical properties of the womb influence behavior for a lifetime. The small, protected characteristics of the womb may explain why certain environmental features are experienced as secure and comforting, including the comfort of a blanket, the relaxation provided by quiet spaces, and the assurance provided by the hugs and embraces of others. These basic needs for security and protection are universal and enduring.

While the womb provides instinctive guidance on features that promote relaxation and safety, other environmental features have been identified as supporting different basic needs. Consider the features typical of kitchens, bathrooms, and bedrooms. Although there are cultural variations, each of these places shares universal characteristics based on its function. Spivak (1973) described such spaces as archetypal. An *archetype* is any object that is deeply rooted in human history and serves as a symbol or model for other objects. According to Spivak, **archetypal places** meet humankind's basic needs for shelter, space, sleeping, mating, grooming, feeding, toileting, playing, competing, working, storing possessions, and meeting with others (Spivak, 1973).

Aspects of Places

Places have different aspects or layers, each influenced by the other (Hamilton, 2004; Barker, 1963). The most obvious aspect of place concerns its physical attributes, location, and the objects and furnishings associated with it. People usually experience physical space through the senses from properties such as temperature, lighting, color, and noise. Many places have natural characteristics that differentiate them, such as proximity to mountains, water, trees, or open spaces.

Affordances

Architects and designers understand the term **affordance** to mean how the design of objects and places can signify their uses. Gibson (1977) coined the term affordance to refer to the perceived characteristics of objects in an environment that intuitively invite certain actions. Affordance is thus an interaction between an object and a person; the object's features suggest its potential or intended purpose, function, and usability.

Consider the affordance of doors. Doors with flat horizontal bars in the middle of the door afford the movement of pushing; those with vertical bars on one side afford the ability to pull, those with round knobs afford pulling and twisting (Masoudi et al., 2019). Chairs offer another example of affordance through their design features such as seat height, size, fabrication material, seating surface, and weight-bearing capacity. There are also affordances in nature. A flat surface boulder about the height of a person's knee naturally invites sitting, particularly on a mountain hike; crevices also afford stepping during rock climbing. In the virtual world, a button on a website is interpreted by the user as an invitation to click.

Distance

Another characteristic of places is their distance from other places. Distances influence daily routines and can be determined by geography as well as by human planning. The distance from one building to the next, from a school to a home, or the distance from an office to the nearest toilet are each a consequence of human design. When considering the design needs of populations, all segments, including older adults, children with disabilities, or individuals with sensory deficits, should be included. Transportation access is another important element of these design considerations (Audirac, 2008).

The Dimensions of Spaces and Universal Design

Designing places so that they are barrier free, accessible, and usable by all is a central precept of *universal design* principles (Ostroff, 2001). The idea of universal design began in the 1950s and has evolved since into a concept known as **design for all**, promoting the idea that spaces *and* products should be designed without the need for **adaptation** by people of different sizes and abilities. The European Union's Stockholm Declaration of 2004 describes design for all as "design for human diversity, social inclusion and equality" (EIDD, 2004). Design features that conform to these ideals include simplicity, flexibility, low physical effort, intuitive use, tolerance for error, and size and space that enable approach and use. Notions of equitable environments that serve diverse populations are constantly evolving, so that other considerations such as cultural appropriateness, and features that promote wellness, participation, and social integration (such as **visitability**), are becoming integrated into universal design thinking (Center for Inclusive Design and Environmental Access, 2023; Steinfeld & Maisel, 2012; see Box 4.1).

BOX 4.1 THE FACTORS THAT MAKE PLACES VISITABLE

What is Visitability?

Visitability is an accessible design approach for new housing based on the idea that anyone should be able to visit, regardless of their ability or need for mobility devices. A social visit requires the ability to get into the house, to pass through interior doorways, and enter a bathroom to use the toilet.

Visitable homes meet three requirements:

- A grade level (zero step) entrance
- Interior doors with a width of at least 32 inches (82 cm)
- An accessible bathroom on the first floor.

Note: Information based on Maisel (2006) and other sources.

In the United States, the Americans with Disability Act (ADA) as amended, creates a legal requirement that prohibits discrimination based on disability in hiring practices or the design of public spaces (Blanck, 2021). It also requires accommodations to enable paid employment by people with disabling conditions.

Considered in the context of design for all, the requirement for accommodations raises interesting social questions about attitudinal barriers toward marginalized social groups. A global movement spurred during the Pandemic of 2020 heightened awareness of the importance of actively promoting diversity, equity, and inclusion in all aspects of society, including in the design of environments.

Too often, diversity is interpreted to mean ethnic or cultural diversity only; but it also pertains to people with disabilities, members of the LGBTQ community, and people of all ages.

Occupational therapy personnel frequently assess home environments for their safety and accessibility. Yet, it seems ethically important for all professionals serving people with disabilities and older adults to view environments from the standpoint of their *design for all* and *visitability* features.

Aging in Place

Accessibility and visibility are often emphasized as factors relevant to older adults because of physical and mental declines associated with age. The term *aging in place* is frequently used to refer to those environmental and social supports necessary for individuals who want to continue living independently in their homes as long as they can safely do so during older adulthood. This may require modifications to their physical space to improve access or mobility within the home, or it can involve assistance with personal care, meal management, and household chores. An interesting qualitative study involving interviews of 121 adults (age 56–92) showed that choice and control of living arrangements were highly important as were feelings of security and familiarity related to homes and communities. The researchers concluded that place was highly important for the subjects because it related it their social relationships, roles, and sense of identity as capable, autonomous adults (Wiles et al., 2012).

Meanings of Places

Objects help to define a place's meaning and shape its physical characteristics. Examples include memorial objects such as gravestones at cemeteries, ancient artifacts displayed at museums, and works of art at galleries. Yet signs and other features can convey symbolic meaning. The study of symbols is called **semiotics**, and the presence of signs, colors, shapes, and objects can communicate shared meaning. Place names are themselves symbols that identify them and their functions, such as stadium, arena, park, or home. A nation's flag outside a large building often symbolizes that activities of some significance occur there, such as those placed outside of courthouses or other government buildings.

Sometimes the meaning of a place is socially constructed and less universal. Places become associated with events and experiences that can give them both individual and collective meaning. Often, historical events are symbolized through statues and other memorials, and thus attain widespread meaning, such as the 9/11 national memorial in New York City. On a smaller scale, most regions and towns have places that convey meaning to the persons living in those areas, even after the structures are gone. Factories, hospitals, asylums, and schools can be closed and replaced by other structures, yet the locations they occupied can remain embedded in the memories of the people who inhabited them. Thus, locations may convey meaning to individuals even if no physical objects or symbols remain there. On a more personal level, places and locations may be meaningful to smaller groups, such as where weddings or fatal accidents have occurred. Places should be viewed from the subjective standpoint of the person occupying them as well as the objective features they possess (Williams, 2014).

Places can also communicate social status. Appleyard (1979) proposed a symbolic communication theory associated with place that emphasized how such locations communicate power and influence through aesthetic components and exclusivity, such as carefully maintained gated entrances. These features can enhance perceived value and boost the self-identity of those living there.

How Places Support and Influence Occupation

In earlier sections, the principles of designing places and spaces for use by all were discussed. Yet, some environments restrict activity because of characteristics totally unrelated to these factors. Extreme temperatures and terrain, lack of water, distance from civilization, and unsafe conditions are some of the physical features of natural environments that preclude habitability (see Figure 4.4). Sometimes danger arises from conflict and hostility, or even the presence of

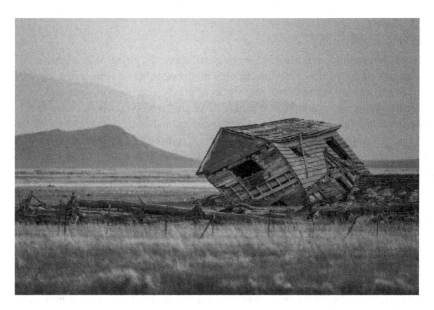

Figure 4.4 Sometimes, places are so remote or barren that they are uninhabitable (Jeff Huth via iStock, used under license)

potentially predatory wildlife. Features that promote and enable activity are those that meet the essential needs of humans, such as safety, access to food and water, and cooperative and supportive group interaction.

Social Capital

The term **social capital** is used to refer to the collective characteristics of places that increase levels of trust, cooperation, interaction (Paldam, 2000). The idea of social capital derives from economics and is intended to reflect differences in the livability or desirability of communities as viewed by the people living in them. Jackson (2020) has proposed a typology that identifies various types of social capital that contribute to the desirability of a community. These include trust, information, coordination, leadership, reputation, and others. Reviews of research by Kawachi and others (Kawachi et al., 2008; Murayama et al., 2012) found evidence of the relationship of social capital to the health of community populations. Places with more social capital are more likely to attract families and businesses because of their perceived safety, which increases the likelihood that people living there will act more sociably.

Environmental Press

Gerontologists Lawton and Nahemow (1973) originated the concept of **environmental press** and competence in their theory of ecological gerontology. Environmental press refers to the physical or psychological demands placed on an individual by characteristics in the environment. The theory proposes that older adults with the competence to satisfactorily overcome environmental barriers of environments, such as social exclusion, will experience better health and well-being.

The extent to which a neighborhood or living setting promotes social interaction through its amenities (gathering places, inhabitants, and social events) is a feature of its press. For older adults, satisfactory habitats must be places that support important transitions, such as retirement and bereavement. Thus, communities with features that promote interaction, cooperation, and a sense of belonging are important.

Virtual Environments

Owing partially to necessities of the pandemic of 2020, virtual meeting platforms multiplied and evolved with features designed to foster convenience and work efficiency. This has influenced the nature of work settings and worker expectations. The evolution of **virtual reality** (VR) for the workplace is an important related development (Wu et al., 2022). Virtual reality has provided a tool that can be used for many purposes through its incorporation of visual, audio, haptic (touch), and kinetic (movement) features. Its use to support interventions for a host of health-related conditions has already been demonstrated through many studies (e.g., Cieślik et al., 2020). The significance of these developments is difficult to overstate, since they change the temporal, physical, location, and transportation requirements of many occupations. Like virtual meeting platforms generally, VR has implications for improving productivity, creativity, and safety, while reducing costs, and providing some beneficial effects on environmental sustainability.

While only limited explorations of the negative consequences of virtual environments have been published in the scholarly literature, there have been calls in the computing industry to address these factors (e.g., Hecht et al., 2021). Some applications create ethical dilemmas on rights to privacy, while others open potential avenues for cyber intrusion or hacking, providing security weaknesses that can lead to unauthorized access to corporate information as well as personal identity theft.

BOX 4.2 THE POINT IS:

- How people use time provides a window into their lifestyles. When time use data is collected for populations, the results provide valuable insights into general social trends, health-related behaviors, and economics.
- Much of behavior is habitual, automatic, and routine. Theories of automaticity maintain that the nervous system is organized to conserve energy and thought for novel situations.
- Behavior is influenced by biological rhythms, with the most important being rest and activity and circadian sleep–wake cycles. Disturbances in the regularity of biological rhythms can have adverse mental and physical health consequences.
- Many diverse physical, social and psychological aspects of places are significant factors in occupational behavior and health. Key concepts of places relate to their social and personal meaning, their accessibility, usability and visitability, and their location.
- Social capital refers to the collective trust and goodwill that promotes interaction and cooperation in communities. There is emerging evidence that there are health benefits to living in places with higher levels of social capital.

References

Adan, A., Archer, S. N., Hidalgo, M. P., Di Milia, L., Natale, V., & Randler, C. (2012). Circadian typology: A comprehensive review. *Chronobiology International, 29*(9), 1153–1175.

Appleyard, D. (1979). The environment as a social symbol: Within a theory of environmental action and perception. *Journal of the American Planning Association,* *45*(2), 143–153.

Arendt, J. (2012). Biological rhythms during residence in polar regions. *Chronobiology international,* *29*(4), 379–394.

Aschoff, J., & Wever, R. (1981). The circadian system of man. In J. Aschoff (Ed.), *Biological rhythms* (pp. 311–331). Springer.

Audirac, I. (2008). Accessing transit as universal design. Journal of Planning Literature, *23*(1), 4–16.

Backman, C. L. (2010). Occupational balance and well-being. In C. Christiansen & E. Townsend (Eds.), *Introduction to occupation: The art and science of living* (pp. 231–249). Slack.

Bargh, J. A. (1994). The four horsemen of automaticity: Intention, awareness, efficiency, and control as separate issues. In R. Wyer & T. Srull (Eds.), *Handbook of social cognition* (pp. 1–40). Lawrence Erlbaum.

Bargh, J. A., & Chartrand, T. L. (1999). The unbearable automaticity of being. *American Psychologist, 54*(7), 462.

Barker, R. G. (1963). On the nature of the environment. *Journal of Social Issues, 19,* 17–38.

Bauman, A., Bittman, M., & Gershuny, J. (2019). A short history of time use research; implications for public health. *BMC Public Health, 19*(2), 1–7.

Beauvalet, J. C., Quiles, C. L., Oliveira, M. A. B. D., Ilgenfritz, C. A. V., Hidalgo, M. P. L., & Tonon, A. C. (2017). Social jetlag in health and behavioral research: A systematic review. *ChronoPhysiology and Therapy, 7,* 19–31.

Blanck, P. (2021). On the importance of the Americans with Disabilities Act at 30. *Journal of Disability Policy Studies,* 10442073211036900.

Blessing, W. W. (2018). Thermoregulation and the ultradian basic rest–activity cycle. *Handbook of clinical neurology, 156,* 367–375.

Center for Inclusive Design and Environmental Access (2023). The goals of universal design. University at Buffalo. www.buffalo.edu/access/help-and-support/topic3/Goa lsofUniversalDesign.html

Christiansen, C. H., & Matuska, K. M. (2006). Lifestyle balance: A review of concepts and research. *Journal of Occupational Science, 13*(1), 49–61.

Christiansen, C.H. (1996). Three perspectives on balance in occupations. In R. Zemke & F. Clark (Eds.), *Occupational science: the evolving discipline* (pp. 431–451). F.A. Davis.

Cieślik, B., Mazurek, J., Rutkowski, S., Kiper, P., Turolla, A., & Szczepańska-Gieracha, J. (2020). Virtual reality in psychiatric disorders: A systematic review of reviews. *Complementary Therapies in Medicine, 52,* 102480.

Cornwell, B., Gershuny, J., & Sullivan, O. (2019). The social structure of time: Emerging trends and new directions. *Annual Review of Sociology, 45*(1), 301–320.

Csikszentmihalyi, M. (1990). Flow: The Psychology of Optimal Experience. Harper & Row.

Eakman, A. M. (2016). A subjectively-based definition of life balance using personal meaning in occupation. *Journal of Occupational Science,* 23(1), 108–127.

Ehlers, C. L., Frank, E., & Kupfer, D. J. (1988). Social zeitgebers and biological rhythms: A unified approach to understanding the etiology of depression. *Archives of General Psychiatry, 45*(10), 948–952.

Ersche, K. D., Lim, T. V., Ward, L. H., Robbins, T. W., & Stochl, J. (2017). Creature of habit: A self-report measure of habitual routines and automatic tendencies in everyday life. *Personality and Individual Differences, 116,* 73–85.

European Institute for Design and Disability (EIDD). (2004). The EIDD Stockholm Declaration. http://dfaeurope.eu/wp-content/uploads/2014/05/stockholm-declaration_english.pdf

Frank, E., Swartz, H. A., & Boland, E. (2022). Interpersonal and social rhythm therapy: An intervention addressing rhythm dysregulation in bipolar disorder. *Dialogues in Clinical Neuroscience, 9*(3), 325–332, https://doi.org/10.31887/DCNS.2007.9.3/efrank

Fritz, H., & Cutchin, M. P. (2016). Integrating the science of habit: Opportunities for occupational therapy. *OTJR: Occupation, Participation and Health,* 36(2), 92–98.

Gardner, B. (2015). A review and analysis of the use of "habit" in understanding, predicting and influencing health-related behaviour. *Health Psychology Review, 9*(3), 277–295.

Gershuny, J. (2011). *Time-use surveys and the measurement of national well-being.* Centre for Time Use Research, University of Oxford, Swansea, UK, Office for National Statistics.

Gershuny, J., Harms, T., Doherty, A., Thomas, E., Milton, K., Kelly, P., & Foster, C. (2020). Testing self-report time-use diaries against objective instruments in real time. *Sociological Methodology, 50*(1), 318–349.

Gibson, J. J. (1977). The theory of affordances. In R. Shaw and J. Bransford (Eds.), *Perceiving, acting, and knowing: Toward an ecological psychology* (pp. 67–82). Lawrence Erlbaum.

Grandin, L. D., Alloy, L. B., & Abramson, L. Y. (2006). The social zeitgeber theory, circadian rhythms, and mood disorders: Review and evaluation. *Clinical Psychology Review, 26*(6), 679–694.

Graybiel, A. M., & Smith, K. S. (2014). Good habits, bad habits. *Scientific American, 310*(6), 38–43.

Hamilton, T. B. (2004). Occupations and places. In C. Christiansen & E. Townsend (Eds.), *Introduction to occupation: The art and science of living* (pp. 173–196). Pearson.

Hecht B, Wilcox L, Bigham JP, Schöning J, Hoque E, De Russis L, Yarosh L, Anjum B, Contractor D, Wu C (2021). It's time to do something: Mitigating the negative impacts of computing through a change to the peer review process. *Association for Computing Machinery (ACM) Future of Computing Blog* (March 29, 2018). https://doi.org/10.48550/arXiv.2112.09544

Ho, E., & Siu, A. M. (2018). Occupational therapy practice in sleep management: A review of conceptual models and research evidence. *Occupational Therapy International,* 1–12. https://doi.org/10.1155/2018/8637498

Hunt, E., & McKay, E. A. (2015). A scoping review of time-use research in occupational therapy and occupational science. *Scandinavian journal of occupational therapy,* 22(1), 1–12.

Jackson, M. O. (2020). A typology of social capital and associated network measures. *Social Choice and Welfare,* 54(2), 311–336.

Kawachi, I., Subramanian, S., Kim, D. (2008). Social Capital and Health. In: Kawachi, I., Subramanian, S., Kim, D. (eds) Social Capital and Health. Springer, New York, NY. https://doi.org/10.1007/978-0-387-71311-3_1

Kielhofner, G. W. (1977). Temporal adaptation. *American Journal of Occupational Therapy, 35*(4), 235–242.

Kleitman, N. (1982). Basic rest–activity cycle—22 years later. *Sleep, 5*(4), 311–317.

Kuhlman, S. J., Craig, L. M., & Duffy, J. F. (2018). Introduction to chronobiology. *Cold Spring Harbor Perspectives in Biology, 10*(9), a033613.

Larson, E., & von Eye, A. (2010). Beyond flow: Temporality and participation in everyday activities. *American Journal of Occupational Therapy, 64*, 152–163.

Lawton, M. P., & Nahemow, L. (1973). Ecology and the aging process. In C. Eisdorfer & M. P. Lawton (Eds.), *The psychology of adult development and aging* (pp. 619–674). American Psychological Association. https://doi.org/10.1037/10044-020

Leland, N. E., Marcione, N., Niemiec, S. L. S., Kelkar, K., & Fogelberg, D. (2014). What is occupational therapy's role in addressing sleep problems among older adults?. *OTJR: Occupation, Participation and Health, 34*(3), 141–149.

Maisel, J. L. (2006). Toward inclusive housing and neighborhood design: A look at visitability. *Community Development, 37*(3), 26–34.

Masoudi, N., Fadel, G. M., Pagano, C. C., & Elena, M. V. (2019). A review of affordances and affordance-based design to address usability. In *Proceedings of the Design Society: International Conference on Engineering 1*(1), 1353–1362. Cambridge University Press.

Meyer, A. (1922). The philosophy of occupational therapy. *Archives of Occupational Therapy, 1*(1), 1–10.

Mistlberger, R. E., & Skene, D. J. (2004). Social influences on mammalian circadian rhythms: Animal and human studies. *Biological Reviews, 79*(3), 533–556.

Mistlberger, R. E., & Skene, D. J. (2005). Nonphotic entrainment in humans? *Journal of Biological Rhythms, 20*(4), 339–352.

Monk, T. H., Kupfer, D. J., Frank, E., & Ritenour, A. M. (1991). The social rhythm metric (SRM): Measuring daily social rhythms over 12 weeks. *Psychiatry Research, 36*(2), 195–207.

Murayama, H., Fujiwara, Y., & Kawachi, I. (2012). Social capital and health: A review of prospective multilevel studies. *Journal of Epidemiology, 22*(3), 179–187.

OECD (2023), Time Use by County. Statistics database, Stats.oecd.org (accessed on March 22, 2023).

Offer, S., & Schneider, B. (2011). Revisiting the gender gap in time-use patterns: Multitasking and well-being among mothers and fathers in dual-earner families. *American Sociological Review, 76*(6), 809–833.

Ostroff, E. (2001). Universal design: The new paradigm. In W. Preiser & E. Ostroff (Eds.), *Universal design handbook* (pp. 1.3–1.12). McGraw-Hill.

Paldam, M. (2000). Social capital: One or many? Definition and measurement. *Journal of Economic Surveys, 14*(5), 629–653.

Pemberton, S., & Cox, D. L. (2015). Synchronisation: Co-ordinating time and occupation. *Journal of Occupational Science, 22*(3), 291–303.

Pyatak, E. A., Carandang, K., Rice Collins, C., & Carlson, M. (2022). optimizing occupations, habits, and routines for health and well-being with lifestyle redesign®: A synthesis and scoping review. *The American Journal of Occupational Therapy, 76*(5). 7605205050.

Roenneberg, T., Foster, R. G., & Klerman, E. B. (2022). The circadian system, sleep, and the health/disease balance: A conceptual review. *Journal of Sleep Research, 31*(4), e13621.

Roenneberg, T., Pilz, L. K., Zerbini, G., & Winnebeck, E. C. (2019). Chronotype and social jetlag: A (self-)critical review. *Biology*, *8*(3), 54. https://doi.org/10.3390/biology8030054

Slagle, E. C. (1922). Training aides for mental patients. *Archives of Occupational Therapy*, *1*(1), 11–18.

Spivak, M. (1973). Archetypal place. Architectural Forum, *140*(3), 44–49.

Steinfeld, E., & Maisel, J. (2012). *Universal design: Creating inclusive environments*. John Wiley & Sons.

Thönes, S., & Oberfeld, D. (2015). Time perception in depression: A meta-analysis. *Journal of Affective Disorders*, *175*, 359–372.

Vagni, G., & Cornwell, B. (2018). Patterns of everyday activities across social contexts. *Proceedings of the National Academy of Sciences*, *115*(24), 6183–6188.

Wagman, P., & Håkansson, C. (2019). Occupational balance from the interpersonal perspective: A scoping review. *Journal of Occupational Science*, *26*(4), 537–545.

Wagman, P., Håkansson, C., & Jonsson, H. (2015). Occupational balance: A scoping review of current research and identified knowledge gaps. *Journal of Occupational Science*, *22*(2), 160–169.

Wiles, J. L., Leibing, A., Guberman, N., Reeve, J., & Allen, R. E. (2012). The meaning of "aging in place" to older people. *The Gerontologist*, *52*(3), 357–366.

Williams, D. R. (2014). Making sense of "place": Reflections on pluralism and positionality in place research. *Landscape and Urban Planning*, *131*, 74–82.

Wu, J., Rajesh, A., Huang, Y. N., Chhugani, K., Acharya, R., Peng, K., ... & Mangul, S. (2022). Virtual meetings promise to eliminate geographical and administrative barriers and increase accessibility, diversity and inclusivity. *Nature Biotechnology*, *40*(1), 133–137.

Yerxa, E. J. (2002). Habits in context: A synthesis, with implications for research in occupational science. *OTJR: Occupation, Participation and Health*, *22*(1_suppl), 104S–110S.

Yokying, P., Sangaroon, B., Sushevagul, T., & Floro, M. S. (2016). Work–life balance and time use: Lessons from Thailand. *Asia-Pacific Population Journal*, *31*(1), 87–107.

Zaki, N. F., Yousif, M., BaHammam, A. S., Spence, D. W., Bharti, V. K., Subramanian, P., & Pandi-Perumal, S. R. (2019). Chronotherapeutics: Recognizing the importance of timing factors in the treatment of disease and sleep disorders. *Clinical Neuropharmacology*, *42*(3), 80–87.

Zuurbier, L. A., Luik, A. I., Hofman, A., Franco, O. H., Van Someren, E. J., & Tiemeier, H. (2015). Fragmentation and stability of circadian activity rhythms predict mortality: The Rotterdam study. *American Journal of Epidemiology 18*, *1*(1), 54–63.

Chapter 5

Sociocultural Influences on Occupation

Introduction

Historically, the development of the profession of occupational therapy emerged through various **sociocultural** influences, including the onset of World War I, the emphasis on the need for humane practices in asylums (moral treatment), and the recognition of the curative properties of occupations (Christiansen & Haertl, 2019). Events and philosophies of the time influenced how occupational therapy started, and the concepts it was built on. Examples included the value placed on hand-made items, crafts, and a concern related to the treatment of those with mental illness. These temporal and sociocultural influences impacted not only the emergence and growth of the profession, but also the daily patterns, habits, roles, routines, environment, and occupational choices made by people in every culture.

The time, locale, norms, and practices within a culture or social group influence the occupations chosen and how they are manifested. For instance, the morning mealtime routine may look very different for a single mother in New York City as compared to a mother in rural Uganda. Familial and cultural norms, habits, and routines influence a person's occupational patterns and engagement. These occupations are further impacted by the sociocultural environment. Daily, these influences surround people through their family and friends, and in the larger society in which they live.

Sociocultural influences on occupation occur on a micro level (e.g., the social influences of family and immediate peer group), a meso level (in communities), and at the macro, or population level (influencing ethnic and national groups) (see Figure 5.1).

These influences affect the environments in which occupations take place along with their **occupational forms**. David Nelson (1988, 1997) introduced the term "occupational form" which was later expanded upon by Nelson and Jepson (2003) as the following:

DOI: 10.4324/9781003242185-5

ENVIRONMENT

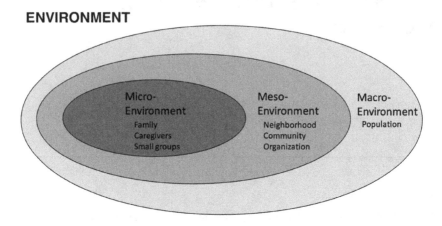

Figure 5.1 Sociocultural influences on occupation

> *Occupational form is the objective set of physical and sociocultural circum-*
> *stances, external to the person, at a particular time. The occupational form*
> *guides, structures or suggests what is done by a person.*
>
> (Nelson & Jepson, 2003, p. 90)

Nelson and Jepson emphasized that dimensions of occupational form include
the physical dimensions such as the texture, sound, weight, size, and temporal/
time aspects of an occupation, as well as the sociocultural dimensions such as
norms, roles, social, and cultural influences. Each of these dimensions impacts
not only occupational choice, but also what an occupation may look like and
how people engage in that occupation. For instance, the occupation of dance
(see Figure 5.2) may take on many occupational forms. In some cultures, the use
of elaborate costumes and instruments such as drums or guitar are an integral
part of the dance. In other cultures, dance may take on the form of the use of
a boom box (hand-held stereo) and a sidewalk along the street, such as often
used in break dancing. Thus, daily occupations are heavily influenced by social
groups, and the culture in which people live. This chapter presents an overview
of sociocultural influences on what and how individuals engage in occupations,
a discussion of **occupational development**, the influences of peer and social
groups, and consideration of how society deems what occupational practices are
acceptable within prevailing sociocultural norms and contexts.

Social Cognition and Occupation

In addition to the sociocultural influences on the form of an occupation, human
doing is shaped not only through personal experiences, but also through watching and participating with others in daily activities. The concept of **agency** refers

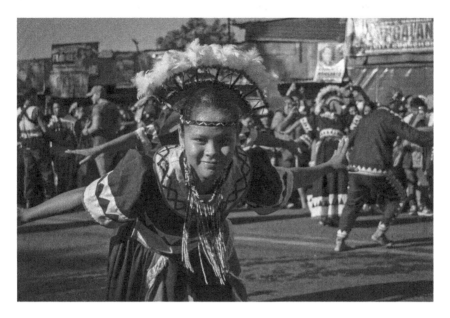

Figure 5.2 The occupation of dance takes on various cultural forms (photo Stephanie Encate, Unsplash)

to an individual's capacity to make personal choices and act upon those choices. Agency influences a person's actions and what they choose to do. Psychologist Albert Bandura, the developer of **social cognitive theory**, wrote "the power to originate actions for given purposes is the key feature of personal agency" (Bandura, 2001, p. 6). He further defined human agency as involving the capacity to influence the self and others. This agency contributes to self-determinism and self-efficacy which, as discussed previously in the book, influence personal identity and meaning. According to Bandura (1989), a person's beliefs about their capacity to act (self-efficacy) influences their thoughts, motivations, and actions.

Bandura's discussion of agency was integral to his development of social learning and social cognitive theory, which suggests that learning occurs in a social context through interactions between the person, environment, and subsequent behavior. These elements later influenced the development of many of the occupation-based models discussed in Chapter 7. Key assumptions of social cognitive theory as presented by Cole and Tufano (2020) include:

- People learn by observing others
- Learning is an internal process

- People are motivated to achieve goals
- People regulate and adjust their own behavior
- Positive and negative reinforcement may have an indirect effect on behavior.

Foundational concepts of social cognitive theory assert that attention, retention, reproduction, and motivation are key to social learning through observation. An individual attends to and selectively observes a given action (attention), retains the information through conceptualization (retention), repeats the action or behavior (reproduction), and through motivation continues to practice and refine the action (Institute for the Scholarship of Assessment, Learning and Teaching, 2014). Thus, people's actions and involvement in occupations are influenced through social observations and the culture in which they live.

Occupational Development and Early Influences on Occupation

People evolve in their choices and occupational patterns via natural development through interaction with others and the environment. Occupational development refers to:

> Change over the life span; development may be a systematic progression of growth and maturation for participation in a repertoire of occupations related to age; or development may be shaped by life circumstances that require an unexpected life path.
>
> (Christiansen & Townsend, 2010a, p. 420)

Throughout the lifespan individuals are influenced through environmental and social interactions that impact occupational development and performance. Humphry (2002) created the Model of Developmental Processes, which includes four key concepts of occupational development: (a) intentional actions, (b) mechanisms for generating occupational behaviors, (c) **sociocultural niche** (children are naturally drawn to culturally relevant occupations), and (d) engagement in occupation as a condition for developmental changes. In addition to the importance of modeling, as discussed within social cognitive theory, Humphry's Model of Developmental Processes was influenced by dynamic systems theory and emphasized intention as crucial to the development of occupation. Such intention involves interest in the behavior of others, along with environmental opportunities for solo and interactional engagement in occupation. Humphery stressed that human activity is not generated from the individual, but is socially constructed and culturally determined (Humphry, 2005).

Humphry used mothering as an example of a role that provides daily routines and opportunities for the development of occupation. For instance, a morning feeding routine followed by a mother talking to her baby and making eye contact involves both the mother and infant. These interactions occur through a joint occupational opportunity often referred to as **co-occupation**, which is defined by Humphry and Thigpen-Beck (1998) as an activity where "the occupational performance of one member depends on the occupational performance of another" (p. 897). Thus, the interactional nature of the activity, such as the morning feeding routine of an infant, influences the occupation. Dickie et al. (2006) emphasized the transactional nature of occupations as involving the physical, social, and cultural context in which the occupation occurs. In the previous example, the infant is influenced not only by the mother–child interaction but also by the environment within which the feeding routine takes place. In some cultures, nursing a baby is often done in a private or semi-private setting, whereas in other cultures, more public expressions of nursing are common. This co-occupation (nursing) may take on many forms and influences development.

Humphry (2016) later extended her work and examples of mother–infant interactions to emphasize the importance of cultural milieu in occupational development. Drawing on examples of multiple researchers, Humphry stressed that, despite expected normal developmental milestones, infant development is influenced by patterns of doing (occupation) within the cultural and environmental setting. Such interactions lay the groundwork for sociocultural influences on occupational patterns and engagement throughout life.

Social Groups, Culture, and Occupation

The concept of co-occupation highlights the interactive nature of occupational engagement. From an early age, people are influenced by their immediate families and social groups along with the greater society around them. Christiansen and Townsend (2010b) distinguished social groups from society, describing the former as a group identified by shared characteristics (e.g., gender, social class, age, etc.), and society as larger communities that often have institutionalized rules, laws, and shared norms or conventions. In addition to the influence of immediate family and their impact on early occupational engagement, peer and social groups often take on increased influence during school age and teen years when identity formation is critical. Psychologist Erik Erickson, known for his work on psychosocial development, stressed the importance of identity development vs. role confusion during the adolescent years (Erickson, 1968). Research indicates that positive peer relationships in adolescence foster identity development and better mental health (Rageliene, 2016). These peer relationships influence occupational choice and occupational engagement (Brennan & Gallagher, 2017; Gallagher et al., 2015).

Christiansen and Townsend (2010b) stressed the importance of active participation within the group to benefit the individual participants and the group

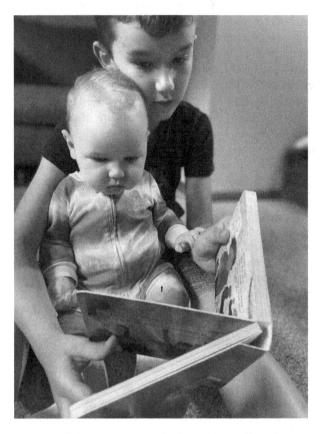

Figure 5.3 Occupational patterns emerge within a family (Photo courtesy of Brianna Haertl)

as a whole. They emphasized that "participation refers to peoples' intentional involvement in circumstances where doing things together can generate a shared identity" (p. 191). As will be discussed later, immediate peer and social groups influence how people spend their time and whether their choices of activities fit within the expectations of the group and society, or whether they are outside societal expectations and norms. For instance, a peer group may involve participation in community sports, often viewed as acceptable and common within societal expectations, or it may be involved in illicit use of drugs and participation in illegal activities, which may be the norm in the immediate peer group, but considered unacceptable within society. The choice of occupations may impact whether an individual and group thrives, or whether a group loses its structure and influence. This collective pattern of occupational choices and engagement influences the future of the group.

Acceptance and Belonging

The previous section discussed the importance of social groups. The influence of groups has biological and evolutionary significance. Within the animal kingdom, the term **herding** is used to describe animals collectively staying together and working towards the benefit of the herd. This concept of herding is necessary for survival. Group behaviors within the herd often align to work towards a common goal (e.g., securing food), and to protect the herd from danger (Marton-Alper et al., 2020).

This same tendency towards the development of group bonds is found in humans. The desire to form and sustain social bonds motivates humans towards social connectedness. Acceptance and belonging are a key function of social groups and participation. Research suggests the importance of meeting the belonging needs of individuals through occupational participation in order to promote health and healing (Gruhl et al., 2020; Renwick & Brown, 1996). Chapter 2 discussed the importance of doing, being, becoming, and belonging and the health-related effects of occupational engagement. Social connectedness and participation serve to meet the human need for belonging.

Fear of **stigma** and **marginalization** may motivate people to conform with sociocultural norms in order to belong, yet historically some groups (e.g., those with disabilities, those of a certain race or class) have experienced collective discrimination and marginalization. Such marginalization may also impact an individual's fear of being stigmatized and influence their activity choices, such as in the case of someone with serious mental health symptoms choosing not to reach out for help. According to the American Psychiatric Association (2021), stigma may lead people to avoid reaching out for help so as not to be classified with those who have mental illness, as they fear the differential treatment they perceive to be associated with being labeled as a member of that group.

The Need to Belong

The innate need for human belonging often influences the choices people make about daily activities to fit in with the social group and greater society. Baumeister and Leary (1995) asserted that humans need close and satisfying social connections. They proposed that this need to belong includes the need to connect with others and that such interpersonal bonds should have a harmonious and sustainable nature in order to meet belongingness needs. This social connection goes beyond a casual affiliation to a more relational context. Once social bonds are formed, there may be a reluctance to discontinue them. Therefore, at times social connections may continue even when the shared occupations or nature of the relationship may not, in societal terms, be in the best interest of the person. Thus, personal social connections have a significant influence on daily habits, roles, routines, and occupational choice.

In addition to the contributions of the psychological and social sciences on theories of belonging, within occupational science and occupational therapy, belonging is viewed as an integral aspect of personal health and well-being (e.g., Wilcock, 1998, 2007). Whereas Wilcock originally wrote of the importance of doing, being and becoming (Wilcock 1998), she later included belonging as an integral part of her dimensions of occupation and health (Hitch et al., 2014; Wilcock, 2007). Renwick (2014) discussed an expanded view of belonging to include *physical belonging*, *social belonging*, and *community belonging*. This broadened view is part of the BBB (Being–Belonging–Becoming) Quality of Life Framework. Within this framework, physical belonging refers to the environmental or physical aspects of the setting in which belonging occurs (e.g., a home, workplace, community). Social belonging involves the immediate social connections with family members, friends, and daily life groups such as work, communities of faith, or a club. Community belonging involves the social connections within the broader community such as with health and social services, parks, and community connections. Each of these types of belonging fills a human need to feel accepted and belong within both the immediate environment, social groups, and the larger community and societal connections in which one engages in throughout life. Such connections may fit into the norms and rules of society, or may deviate from social expectations and be considered **maladaptive** or unacceptable. The next section discusses what is considered adaptive or maladaptive behavior and the concept of **non-sanctioned occupations**.

Maladaptive and Non-Sanctioned Occupations

In recent years within occupational science, literature has explored the concept of maladaptive or non-sanctioned occupations (e.g., Twinley, 2012). Using the term maladaptive could be thought of as judgmental but may be used to discern occupations that are harmful to self, others, or society. Yet categorization of occupations that do or do not fit into the norms of a social group or culture may change over time. For instance, decades ago the heavy tattooing of bodies (sometimes referred to as body art), was rare and outside the norm of many industrialized nations or cultures. Yet tattoos extend back thousands of years and are again more mainstream in present day societies throughout the world. Thus, norms and sociocultural influences change through time.

In addition, the concept of maladaptive infers a societal view on what is considered adaptive. For instance, persons with personality disorder often resort to self-harming behaviors that do not fit into societal norms of healthy behaviors (Potvin et al., 2019). One such action is cutting. Haertl (2019) asserted that cutting could be a behavior, habit, or occupation depending on the circumstances. Cutting may fit the definition of "behavior" in order to "release" anxiety or pain, and if repeated over time it may develop into a habit. Yet in instances of the phenomenon of "cutting parties" it may take on the form of an actual occupation with rituals and socialization with others. Thus, the context in which an action occurs affects our understanding of the action. Further, such actions are often learned from peer groups, yet may also occur through one's own volition. In addition, while cutting is often viewed as maladaptive, if a person with a mental health condition has a history of abuse, the use of cutting may release anxiety and frustration in an attempt to avoid suicide, and one could argue that such cutting is an adaptation of self-preservation. These behaviors are outside of the sociocultural norms and may be considered "non-sanctioned."

The term "non-sanctioned occupations," was introduced by Kiepek et al. (2019) to refer to occupations that, within historically and culturally bound contexts, tend to be viewed as "unhealthy, illegal, immoral, abnormal, undesired, unacceptable, and/or inappropriate" (p. 341). The authors proposed that expanding occupational science scholarship to include non-sanctioned occupations would extend knowledge of human engagement in daily life. The concept of "sanctioned" in non-sanctioned occupations refers to that which is deemed acceptable in a given group, religion, society, or culture. Failure to conform with written or unwritten rules and norms may result in ostracization or criminalization.

As previously discussed, the context in which non-sanctioned occupations occurs must be considered prior to categorizing something as healthy, unhealthy, adaptive, or maladaptive. For instance, in most societal norms, theft would be considered as an unhealthy harmful behavior, not only to the individuals involved, but also to the greater society. Yet if put in the context of someone in an area of heavy natural disaster who steals from a store with an open wall in order to feed their family, one may consider this from a different lens, as concepts of acceptable, adaptive and sanctioned become more conditional. Thus, the understanding of non-sanctioned occupations must consider the context of the activity within a larger societal lens. In systems of oppression peaceful protests may be seen as appropriate, but violent acts may be socially sanctioned only in exteme conditions. In addition, the understanding of the reasoning and context surrounding occupations that may be harmful (e.g., heavy alcohol and drug use that leads to crime or severed relationships), can elucidate approaches that individually and systematically address underlying issues necessary for promoting the health and well-being of individuals and society. Environmental context must also be considered in order to fully respond to areas that may need to be addressed.

Environmental Influences on Social Groups

In addition to interpersonal connections, the external environment affects social groups and occupational participation. According to the OT Practice Framework 4th edition, environmental factors include natural and built environments along with technology and products, physical and emotional supports, attitudes (customs, practices, and norms), and social systems and policies (American Occupational Therapy Association, 2020). These factors may create occupational opportunities or barriers to participation for individuals and groups. In addition to social learning, the environment influences our occupational engagement.

As mentioned in Chapter 4, Murray et al. (1938) theorized the importance of environmental factors that influence action. He termed this "environmental press." Gerontologist M. P. Lawton (1983) extended concepts of environmental press to aging adults and asserted that the differences between the individual (person) and the environmental pressures and variables often require adaptation. Thus, environmental and individual variables influence a person's actions and how they are completed. For instance, a woman in a wheelchair with a spinal cord injury may have to adapt a kitchen used prior to the accident in order to have the capacity to complete cooking tasks. This task would be further affected if there are social influences such as family members who can provide support and assistance with the kitchen tasks. These environmental and social influences on occupation begin at birth and extend throughout the lifespan.

If the environment has the necessary elements and supports such as in a well-equipped school with a low student to teacher ratio and programming to facilitate learning for all, student engagement and learning may thrive. Yet in instances with low environmental supports and programming, meeting the overall learning goals of the school and pupils may be compromised. This environmental impact may occur on a micro (e.g., familial) level, a meso (group) level, or the macro (population) level. Understanding environmental influences on groups and communities is important in occupational science and occupational therapy.

For instance, during the Covid-19 pandemic, there were several environmental shifts in occupational opportunities for groups. Sporting events ceased, schools, churches, temples, and community groups went to online formats, and in-person social connections with friends and family were greatly reduced. Many adapted with the emergence of vaccinations and people were again able to get out in their communities and gather in groups. Yet some groups had lasting change and occupational shifts, such as school programs that reverted to hybrid formats, workplaces that chose to remain hybrid, and houses of worship that conducted services both in person and online. During this time many businesses and colleges closed due to the negative economic impact of the pandemic on these groups and institutions. Thus, environmental influences affect not only the individual choice and engagement in occupation, but also the collective occupations shared within groups and how these groups and institutions change through time. This environmental influence will be further discussed in Chapter 6, in relation to occupational justice, that environmental conditions within a society affect opportunities for occupational choice and engagement. For instance, people in geographic areas experiencing war, poverty, or natural disaster often have limitations in time and resources that affect their ability to participate in everyday occupations.

Cultural Influences on Occupation

There are a number of definitions of culture. While the term often refers to a particular ethnic group or geographical region, present day **conceptualizations** extend beyond this to include social groups, norms, and practices. The Oxford Dictionary (2022) defines culture as "The customs, arts, social institutions, and achievements of a particular nation, people, or other social group." Thus, culture is broadened beyond ethnicity and may discern a way of life, norms, and practices of a particular group. This includes language and communication patterns within a culture such as in the differing languages and dialects used within a country, or the terminology used in a profession such as occupational therapy. These patterns of communication influence values, worldviews, and the understanding people have of their relationships, group affiliations, and the meaning they place on daily activities. As discussed earlier, such concepts of personal meaning influence identity, occupational choices, and occupational engagement.

It is important to note that culture may be used to consider the influences of a group or society and may also be applied at the individual level. For instance, culture at a societal level includes the practices and beliefs of a particular group or geographical region. Culture at the individual level crosses many groups and categorizations such as race, gender, ethnicity, religious affiliation etc. (Nastasi et al., 2017). This intersection of membership in cultural groups can influence an individual's development, worldview and occupational engagement throughout life. Additionally, cultural norms and practices help people construct systems of meaning, knowledge and action (Nastasi & Hitchcock, 2015; Nastasi et al., 2017). The meaning and value of a particular group influences how a person engages in daily activities. For instance, Cai, an 18-year-old adolescent male, may highly value his Hmong heritage and engage in many community cultural events. Yet, at the same time, Cai may choose not to participate in the familial religious events. Therefore, although there may be numerous cultural influences on an individual, differences will exist based on the value and meaning associated with each activity within different subgroups.

Culture and Occupational Choice

Concepts of occupational choice extend back to the 1950s when Blau et al. (1956) discussed the individual, psychological, social, and economic factors that influence the choice of a vocation. They created a conceptual framework of occupational choice, emphasizing individual and societal factors in career selection. They emphasized that, in addition to cultural influences, an individual must have knowledge of the occupational opportunities available at the time a vocational choice is made. The environment in which one makes the choice and the sociocultural influences impact the career one selects. If an individual doesn't have knowledge of a particular vocation, they may not seek the education needed to pursue that career. For instance, many students indicate that by chance they learned of the field of occupational therapy, either through exposure at a work site, a relative who experienced OT, or a friend that planned on attending OT school. Through exposure to the opportunity, these OT students then went on to pursue the career. Without greater knowledge of professions, a person's choices are diminished. Similarly, the occupations that people are exposed to through their cultural affiliations can inform their occupational choices in all areas of daily activity, as described below.

Within occupational science and therapy, the concept of occupational choice has been extended to refer to individual choices in daily activities. The occupational choices made are influenced by sociocultural groups and thus must be considered through a cultural lens (Brennan & Gallagher, 2017; Galvaan, 2015). Further, the cultures in which one affiliates may influence the meaning ascribed to an occupation. According to Wilcock and Townsend (2019), the values attributed to an occupation are influenced by sociopolitical and cultural determinants. For some individuals, lawn care and homemaking may be considered informal work, yet for others, these activities are taken on as leisure occupations. In addition, both culture and resources influence occupational choice and engagement. For instance, in the previous example of lawn care and home making, while many include this as part of their daily occupational activities, in some cultures, lawn care, cooking, and other homemaking tasks may be performed by paid workers within the home. This illustrates that cultural context influences occupational choice and meaning.

Culture in Occupational Science and Occupational Therapy

The profession of occupational therapy has long emphasized the importance of culturally compassionate care. Black and Wells (2007) expanded the definition of culture as:

> The sum total of a way of living, including values, beliefs, standards, linguistic expression, patterns of thinking, behavioral norms, and styles of communication that influence the behavior(s) of a group of people (and) is transmitted from generation to generation. It includes demographic variables such as age, gender, and place of residence; status variables such as social, educational, and economic levels and affiliation variables.
>
> Black & Wells, 2007, p. 5)

This expanded view emphasizes the importance of considering not only a client's current cultural status and the many subcultures they belong to, but also the generational influences that impact a client's values, beliefs, and occupational patterns. Thus, an occupational pattern for common daily activities (e.g., grooming or cooking) impacted by the client's culture. For instance, Thein-Lemelson (2015) conducted a **mixed-methods** study of grooming and cultural socialization. Findings suggested that Burmese children are groomed more often than their counterparts in the United States and more in-culture differences exist in Burmese grooming practices than are found in the United States. Therefore, cultural norms and practices can affect how activities of daily living (ADL) and instrumental activities of daily living (IADL) are practiced. Occupational patterns common to a culture are further influenced by the fact that some cultures are more individualistic in nature, and other cultures emphasize collectivist practices that emphasize the interdependence of people. This difference in cultural structure and beliefs impacts not only occupational patterns, but also values and decision making. Huppert et al. (2019) compared children in 13 countries from both individualistic and collectivist societies. The authors found differences in concepts of equity in children raised in collectivist countries as compared to those in countries deemed to have individualistic values. Overall, children in individualistic countries favored equitable distribution related to wealth and merit; however, when empathy was factored in and with respect to disabilities, and the level of injury experienced by an individual was considered, then those in collectivist countries had a greater desire for equity. This suggests that cultural upbringing affects not only a person's occupational choices and patterns, but also a person's underlying philosophical views of the world, which affect decision making and choice.

Cultural Competence

In the past two decades, there has been increasing emphasis on the importance of **cultural competence** in providing health care services. Cultural competence emphasizes knowledge, skills, awareness, attitudes, and processes necessary to equitably serve people from diverse backgrounds (Bean, 2006; Gopalkrishnan, 2019). Frameworks have been developed around the concept of cultural competence in order to guide individuals and organizations in service delivery to diverse populations. Emphasis is placed on training health care providers to provide culturally competent care, yet critics assert that the perspectives used in training are often disproportionately influenced by the Northern Hemisphere and fail to consider power differentials and other dynamics that may exist in different cultures (Gopalkrishnan, 2019).

While cultural competence does emphasize the importance of educating practitioners in providing care to diverse populations, concern is raised over the premise that someone can become totally culturally competent. Gupta (2008) asserted that it "implies that a hypothetical endpoint exists that can be reached by acquiring the right knowledge and skills and attitudes needed to work with people of different cultures" (p. 3). Rather than considering cultural competence as an end point, approaches should be taken to ensure a dynamic partnership between the practitioner and client or between service providers and organizations in order to assure the needs of all individuals and parties are addressed.

As an alternative to culturally competent care, Munoz (2007) proposed the term "culturally responsive caring" to include the importance of mutuality in working with a client. Munoz also emphasized that the education we have about a particular culture may or may not fit with the client. Therefore, a client-centered approach must consider the individual perspectives, culture, worldview, and priorities of the client in the occupational therapy process.

Summary

Throughout their lifespan, individuals are influenced by the groups, communities, and cultures in which they engage. Sociocultural influences on occupational patterns, engagement, and choice occur at the micro (familial and small group), meso (community), and macro (population) levels. This chapter has presented a discussion of the formation of occupational engagement through social learning and occupational development, the importance of societal norms and worldviews on individuals and groups, and the concept of maladaptive and non-sanctioned occupations.

Individuals have an innate need to belong to groups, and marginalization and stigmatization may affect occupational choice. Cultural influences on occupation may occur at the societal level and at the individual level. Culturally responsive caring seeks to understand the culture of the client, and the individual differences and meaning within the environment in which they live (see Box 5.1).

BOX 5.1 THE POINT IS:

- Families and social groups influence occupational choice and engagement throughout the lifespan.
- *Co-occupation* refers to a joint occupational activity in which simultaneous participation influences both the occupational engagement and persons involved.
- The environment influences individual and group participation in occupation.
- A person belongs to multiple cultural groups, each of which uniquely influences occupational choice and participation.

References

American Occupational Therapy Association (AOTA). (2020). Occupational therapy practice framework: Domain and process (4th ed.). *American Journal of Occupational Therapy, 74*(Suppl. 2), 7412410010.

American Psychiatric Association (APA). (2021). *Stigma, prejudice, and discrimination against people with mental illness.* www.psychiatry.org/patients-families/stigma-and -discrimination

Bandura, A. (1989). Human agency in social cognitive theory. *American Psychologist, 44*(9), 1175–1184. https://doi.org/10.1037/0003-066X.44.9.1175

Bandura, A. (2001). Social cognitive theory: An agentic perspective. *Annual Review of Psychology, 52*, 1–26. https://doi.org/10.1146/annurev.psych.52.1.1

Baumeister, R. F., & Leary, M. R. (1995). The need to belong: Desire for interpersonal attachments as a fundamental human motivation. *Psychological Bulletin, 117*(3), 497–529. https://doi.org/10.1037/0033-2909.117.3.497

Bean, R. (2006). *The effectiveness of cross cultural training in the Australian context.* Canberra: Department of Immigration and Cross Cultural Affairs.

Black, R. M., & Wells, S. A. (2007). *Culture and occupation: A model of empowerment in occupational therapy.* AOTA Press.

Blau, P. M., Gustad, J. W., Jessor, R., Parnes, H. S., & Wilcock, R. C. (1956), Occupational choice: A conceptual framework. *Industrial and Labor Relations Review, 9*(4), 531–543.

Brennan, G. J., & Gallagher, M. (2017). Expectations of choice: An exploration of how social context informs gendered occupation. *Irish Journal of Occupational Therapy, 45*(1), 15–27. ISSN: 2398-8819.

Christiansen, C. H., & Haertl, K. L. (2019). A contextual history of occupational therapy. In B. Schell & G. Gillen (Eds.), *Willard & Spackman's occupational therapy: Centennial edition.* (13th ed., pp. 11–42). Lippincott Williams & Wilkins.

Christiansen, C. H., & Townsend, E. A. (2010a). *Introduction to occupation: The art and science of living* (2nd ed.). Pearson.

Christiansen, C. H., & Townsend, E. A. (2010b). The occupational nature of social groups. In C. H. Christiansen, & E. A. Townsend (Eds.), *Introduction to occupation: The art and science of living* (2nd ed., 175–210). Pearson.

Cole, M. B., & Tufano, R. (2020). *Applied theories in occupational therapy: A practical approach.* Slack.

Dickie, V., Cutchin, M. P., & Humphry, R. (2006). Occupation as transactional experience: A critique of individualism in occupational science. *Journal of Occupational Science, 13*(1), 83–93. https://doi.org/10.1080/14427591.2006.9686573

Erickson, E. H. (1968). *Identity youth and crisis.* W. W. Norton.

Gallagher, M. B., Pettigrew, J., & Muldoon, O. (2015), Occupational choice of youth in a disadvantaged community, *British Journal of Occupational Therapy, 78*(10), 622–629. https://doi.org/10.1177/0308022615583065

Galvaan, R. (2015). The contextually situated nature of occupational choice: Marginalised young adolescents' experiences in South Africa. *Journal of Occupational Science, 22*(1), 39–53. https://doi.org/10.1080/14427591.2014.912124

Gruhl, K. L., Boucher, M., & Lacarte, S. (2020). Evaluation of an occupation-based program: Meeting being, becoming and belonging needs. *Australian Journal of Occupational Therapy, 68*, 78–89. https://doi.org/10.1111/1440-1630.12707

Gopalkrishnan, N. (2019). Cultural competence and beyond: Working across culture in dynamic partnerships. *The International Journal of Community and Social Development, 1*(1), 28–41.

Gupta, J. (2008). Reflections of one educatory on teaching cultural competence. *Education SIS Quarterly, 18*, 3.

Haertl, K. L. (2019). *Occupation? Behavior? Habit?: The intersection of self-harm.* Presented at the SSO: USA Annual Research Conference, Kentucky.

Hitch, D., Pepin, G., & Stagnitti, K. (2014). In the footsteps of Wilcock part one: The evolution of doing, being, becoming and belonging. *Occupational Therapy in Healthcare, 28*(3), 231–246. https://doi.org/10.3109/07380577.2014.898114

Humphry, R. (2002). Young children's occupations: Explicating the dynamics of developmental processes. *American Journal of Occupational Therapy, 56*, 171–179. https://doi.org/10.5014/ajot.56.2.171

Humphry, R. (2005). Model of processes transforming occupation: Exploring societal and social influences. *Journal of Occupational Science, 12*(1), 36–44.

Humphry, R. (2016). Joining in, interpretative reproduction, and transformations of occupations: What is "know-how" anyway?, *Journal of Occupational Science, 23*(4), 422–433. https://doi.org/10.1080/14427591.2016.1210000

Humphry, R., & Thigpen-Beck, B. (1998). Parenting values and attitudes: Views of parents and therapists. *American Journal of Occupational Therapy, 52*(10), 825–842. https://doi.org/10.5014/ajot.52.10.835

Huppert, E., Cowell, J. M., Cheng, Y., Contereras-Ibanez, C., Gomez-Sicard, N., Gonzalez-Gadia, L., Huepe, D., Ibanez, A., Lee, K., Mahasneh, R., Malcom-Smith, S., Salas, N., Selcuk, B., Tungodden, B., Wong, A., Zhou, X., & Decety, J. (2019). The development of children's preferences for equality and equity across 13 individualistic and collectivist cultures. *Developmental Science, 22*(2), e12729. https://doi.org/10.1111/desc.12729

Institute for the Scholarship of Assessment, Learning and Teaching (2014). *Social cognitive theory.* Minnesota State University.

Kiepek, N. C., Beagan, B., Rudman, D. L., & Phelan, S. (2019). Silences around occupations framed as unhealthy, illegal and deviant. *Journal of Occupational Science, 3,* 341–353. https://doi.org/10.1080/14427591.2018.1499123

Lawton, M. P. (1983). Environment and other determinants of well-being in older people. *Gerontologist, 23,* 349–357. https://doi.org/10.1093/geront/23.4.349

Marton-Alper, I. Z., Gvirts-Provolovski, H. Z., Nevat, M., & Shmay-Tsoory, S. G. (2020). Herding in human groups is related to highly autistic traits. *Scientific Reports, 10,* Article 17950. https://doi.org/10.1038/s41598-020-74951-8

Munoz, J. (2007). Culturally responsive caring to occupational therapy. *Occupational Therapy International, 14,* 256–280. https://doi.org/10.1002/oti.238

Murray, H. A., Barrett, W. G., & Hamburger, E. (1938). *Explorations in personality.* Oxford University Press.

Nastasi, B. K. & Hitchcock, J. H. (2015). *Mixed methods research and culture-specific interventions: Program design and evaluation.* Sage.

Nastasi, B. K., Arora, P. G., & Varjas, K. (2017). The meaning and importance of cultural construction for global development. *International Journal of School and Educational Psychology, 5*(3), 137–140. https://doi.org/10.1080/21683603.2016.1276810

Nelson, D. L. (1988). Occupation: Form and performance. *American Journal of Occupational Therapy, 42,* 633–641. https://doi.org/10.5014/ajot.42.10.633

Nelson, D. L. (1997). Why the profession of occupational therapy will flourish in the 21st century. The 1996 Eleanor Clark Slagle lecture. *American Journal of Occupational Therapy, 51,* 11–24. https://doi.org/10.5014/ajot.51.1.11

Nelson, D. L., & Jepson, J.-T. (2003). Occupational form, occupational performance, and a conceptual framework for therapeutic occupation. In P. Kramer, J. Hinojosa, & C. B. Royeen (Eds.), *Perspectives in human occupation: Participation in life* (pp. 87–155). Lippincott Williams & Wilkins.

Oxford Dictionary. (2022). Culture. www.lexico.com/en/definition/culture

Potvin, O., Valee, C., Lariviere, N. (2019). Experience of occupations among people living with a personality disorder. *Occupational Therapy International,* Article 9030897. https://doi.org/10.1155/2019/9030897

Rageliene, T. (2016). Links of adolescents identity development and relationship with peers: A systematic literature review. *Journal of the Canadian Academy of Child and Adolescent Psychiatry, 25*(2), 97–105.

Renwick, R. (2014). Fostering and supporting quality of life: Focus on the person in context. In K. Haert (Ed.), *Adults with intellectual and developmental disabilities: Strategies for occupational therapy* (pp. 41–58). AOTA Press.

Renwick, R., & Brown, I. (1996). The centre for health promotion's conceptual approach to quality of life. In R. Renwick, I. Brown, & M. Nager (Eds.), *Quality of life in health promotion and rehabilitation: Conceptual approaches, issues and applications* (pp. 75–86). Sage.

Thein-Lemelson, S. M. (2015). Grooming and cultural socialization: A mixed-method study of caregiving practices in Burma and the United States. *International Journal of Psychology, 50*(1), 37–46. https://doi.org/10.1002/ijop.12119

Twinley, R. (2012). The dark side of occupation: A concept for consideration. *Australian Occupational Therapy Journal, 60*(4), 301–303. https://doi.org/.1111/1440-1630 .12026

Wilcock, A. A. (1998). Reflections on doing, being and becoming. *Canadian Journal of Occupational Therapy, 65*, 248–256. https://doi.org/10.1177/000841749806500501

Wilcock, A. A. (2007). Occupation and health: Are they one and the same? *Journal of Occupational Science, 14*(1), 3–8. https://doi.org/10.1080/14427591.2007.9686577

Wilcock, A. A., & Townsend, E. A. (2019). Occupational justice. In B. A. Schell & G. Gillen (Eds.), *Willard and Spackman's occupational therapy* (13th ed., pp. 643–659). Lippincott Williams & Wilkins.

Chapter 6

Occupational Justice
Occupation Viewed from a Social Lens

Introduction

Principles of social justice date back to the 19th century and refer to social equity, or often inequity, in terms of distribution of wealth, privilege, and opportunity. Political, social, and economic practices influence justice and the individual vs. collective nature of society. In the 1990s, the concept of **occupational justice** emerged to denote the importance of occupational opportunities available in society in order to have meaningful engagement in occupations necessary for health and well being. Wilcock and Townsend (2000) initially presented the concept as complementary to social justice in referring to justice regarding what people do, the opportunities they have, and the conditions for living. The concept evolved from a workshop in 2000 held in Australia. The workshop dialogue about the idea of unjust barriers to occupation prompted similar conversations in several other countries, soon extending to the role of occupational therapy in addressing occupational inequities in all populations (Wilcock & Townsend, 2019). Since then, literature in occupational science and occupational therapy has evolved and frameworks of occupational justice have expanded to include moral, ethical, and civil issues relevant to society.

Evolving Definitions

Whereas occupational justice was originally conceptualized under the broad category of social justice, recent frameworks describe a more complex view of how occupational justice applies to social values and practices (e.g., Wilcock & Townsend, 2019). Wilcock and Townsend (2000) originally described occupational justice as "equitable opportunity and resources to enable people's engagement in meaningful occupations" (p. 85). They expanded on this definition to align social and occupational justice through noting that justice and equity are important factors underlying:

DOI: 10.4324/9781003242185-6

- Opportunities to participate in meaningful occupation
- Meeting human needs as occupational beings to participate in work
- Meeting important spiritual needs of individuals and communities
- Satisfying socially determined mental, physical, social, and spiritual needs
- Distributing adequate resources through political and organizational systems.

According to Townsend and Wilcock (2004), occupational justice also has implications for client-centered occupational therapy. While the basic principles of occupational justice have remained consistent, definitions have broadened and expanded over time. For example, Stadnyk et al. (2010) described occupational justice as focusing on "meaningful and purposeful occupations (tasks and activities) that people want to do, need to do, and can do considering their personal and situational circumstances" (p. 331). This definition was further expanded by Wilcock and Hocking (2015), to emphasize that opportunities for personal development and social inclusion were explicit elements of the concept. Additional terminology discussed in the next section is relevant to the study of occupational justice and lays the foundation for the remainder of the chapter.

Terminology

There are several related terms associated with occupational justice that aid in the understanding of the concept. While the following terms are not meant to be all inclusive, they help the reader understand major principles of occupational justice as it has evolved in the literature. **Occupational determinants** are factors such as the national and international policies, type of economy, policy values, and cultural values that contribute to conditions of occupational justice (Stadnyk et al., 2010). For instance, people are born into a certain culture, economic situation, and political system. Such systems affect personal occupational opportunity and influence the distribution of wealth in the society in which they live (see Figure 6.1).

Occupational injustice refers to the denial (or limitation) of occupational opportunity that may result from being deprived of access to meaningful occupations or forced to participate in unchosen occupations. Durocher et al. (2014) conducted a scoping review that revealed five forms of occupational injustice outlined in the literature; specific examples of occupational injustice will be presented later in the chapter.

- *Occupational Apartheid:* Situations in which occupations are granted or denied to individuals based on characteristics such as gender, age, race, nationality, sexuality, etc. (Kronenberg & Pollard, 2005)

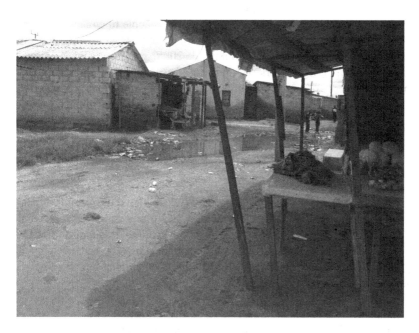

Figure 6.1 Social determinants of health influence occupational opportunities and occupational justice. This village has little infrastructure and when it rains flooding impacts the community and may cause disintegration of housing (photo courtesy of Paula Rabaey)

- *Occupational Deprivation:* "a state of preclusion from engagement in occupations of necessity and/or meaning due to factors that stand outside the immediate control of the individual" (Whiteford, 2000, p. 201)
- *Occupational Marginalization:* People are not given the opportunity for occupational participation or to exert choice and decision making, this may occur through norms, societal practices, or even occupational apartheid (Stadnyk et al., 2010)
- *Occupational Alienation:* Refers to "prolonged experience of disconnectedness, isolation, emptiness, lack of a sense of identity, a limited or confined expression of spirit, or a sense of meaninglessness" (Townsend & Wilcock, 2004, p. 80)
- *Occupational Imbalance:* The allocation of time use that may occur when an individual spends too much time in a specific occupation or area of occupation at the expense of other occupations (Stadnyk et al., 2010). For instance, if a person has to work so much in paid employment that they lack time for childrearing and spending time with their children and family.

The above terms relate to how occupational injustice may occur. The final concept, **occupational rights**, refers to "the right of all people to engage in meaningful occupations that contribute positively to their own well-being and the well-being of their communities" (Hammell, 2008, p. 62). As occupational therapists, it is important to work within the profession and in multidisciplinary communities in order to assure the rights of clients and populations are served to engage in meaningful occupation. Later in the chapter, practical applications of occupational justice to occupational therapy will be discussed.

Key Principles and Emerging Frameworks

Principles

For occupational therapists to apply concepts of occupational justice, it is important to understand the foundational principles and frameworks. Occupational justice emphasizes the rights of individuals to have equitable opportunities for meaningful occupation in order to have participation, choice, and engagement in everyday activity. Stadnyk et al. (2010) identified foundational beliefs of occupational justice to include the following:

- Humans are occupational beings
- Humans are individual autonomous agents in participation
- Occupational participation is interdependent and contextual
- Occupational participation is a determinant of health and quality of life.

Within these beliefs, the authors identified the empowerment, inclusion, and enablement of diversity as important principles of occupational justice. Collectively, these principles are aimed at working towards an occupationally just society that considers the needs of individuals and groups and promotes choice as an opportunity for meaningful engagement. Concepts of occupational justice seek to embrace the differences in occupation, yet provide equitable opportunities for participation.

Frameworks

Occupational justice frameworks consider not only the facets of occupational justice described above, but also how occupational therapists may work toward meaningful change. Central to theory underlying occupational justice frameworks is the concept that human empowerment is attained through occupation and is dependent on the power relations that shape occupational engagement (Wilcock & Townsend, 2019). Townsend and Wilcock (2004) advocated for client-centered activism to promote occupational justice. They asserted the need for the development of research and educational strategies to enact meaningful change. The authors suggested that action research, participatory evaluation techniques (e.g., the Canadian Occupational Performance Measure (COPM) (CAOT, 2022), and evaluation of community-based needs would provide increased insights as to where occupational therapy could work to promote occupational justice.

Wilcock and Townsend (2019) emphasized that their framework applies to multiple levels of service provision. At the *individual action level* therapists may work individually to promote occupation-based programs, and identify potential actions to support engagement in occupation. At the *group action level* partnerships are made with advocacy and other groups (e.g., the socially disadvantaged or marginalized, justice-based local organizations etc.) in order to work for community change, and at the *collective action* level, consideration is given to global alliances for collective change through partnerships with larger entities such as international groups, non-governmental organizations, or the World Federation of Occupational Therapists. Within this collective action, Wilcock and Townsend (2019) presented the *Occupational Justice and Health Questionnaire*, which is a tool to identify whether communities are able to meet the occupational rights of individuals. The authors suggested that occupational therapists develop occupational justice/injustice checklists in order to identify areas of injustice and potential action for change.

Townsend and Whiteford (2005) extended the initial occupational justice concepts and framework to develop a participatory occupational justice framework to facilitate social inclusion through raising awareness and addressing occupational injustice. The **Participatory Occupational Justice Framework (POJF)** includes six interlocking non-linear components addressing processes for environmental and social change along with consideration for implementation of client-specific services. The interlocking circles of the participatory occupational justice framework are as follows:

- Analyze occupational injustices
- Evaluate strengths, resources, and challenges
- Implement and evaluate services
- Negotiate program designs, outcomes, and evaluations
- Negotiate a justice framework
- Analyze and coordinate resources.

The authors asserted that the overlapping processes above are non-linear and thus different areas of work may involve different stages of the framework. For instance, when working with occupational therapy students in a refugee program in the United States, it was necessary for the author involved (KH) to develop rapport and establish a relationship with the organization, its staff, and the clients served prior to engaging in any of the processes above. Once engaged with the site, evaluations could take place, along with an analysis of the strengths and needs, and then an overarching justice framework could be developed along with a plan for collaboration. Within other services, it may be important to start with another process first and thus contextual considerations must be included in applying the framework.

Gail Whiteford and colleagues (Whiteford et al., 2018) presented case examples of the POJF and affirmed its non-linearity, yet asserted that a natural starting point for addressing occupational injustice was to raise awareness of the injustice itself. Those authors also recommended that a natural closing point for justice work should include an agreement on next steps and strategies for long-term sustainability. Again, context is important as occupational justice work may include the evaluation and recommendation phase, or may also include justice actions to address areas identified in the evaluation. The authors depicted this reimagined version of POJF to discuss collaborative processes for justice. Their model includes a center circle with the words "collaborative enabling processes" with arrows moving outward towards six circles including:

- Raise a consciousness of occupational injustice
- Engage collaboratively with partners
- Mediate agreement on a plan
- Strategic resource funding
- Support implementation and continuous evaluation
- Inspire advocacy for sustainability or closure.

While the authors acknowledge non-linearity, their six processes appear to have a natural order; however, given the dynamic nature of community work, there are often changes in plans or processes that may necessitate re-evaluation and change of plan. See Box. 6.1 as an example of occupational justice work completed in Uganda.

BOX 6.1 OCCUPATION IN ACTION: OCCUPATIONAL JUSTICE IN DEVELOPING COUNTRIES

In the service of promoting environments where the health-related benefits of purposeful engagement are available to all, occupational therapists may work to change underlying structures that limit or restrict participation. Associate Professor Paula Rabaey, Ph.D., MPH, OTR/L works with interprofessional teams and students in a number of countries to address issues of disability awareness, access, and barriers to occupational engagement. She also works to empower community members and caregivers to support children with disabilities. An integral part of this global work is collaboration with local partners, shared assessment of needs, and development of a plan.

An example is her work with the Spoon Foundation, a Non-Govermental Organization (NGO) based in Portland, Oregon whose mission is to nourish the world's most vulnerable children. Dr. Rabaey worked with the Foundation to develop a special feeding chair that may be used to enhance mealtime participation for children with disabilities who are unable to feed, eat, or engage in mealtime with their caregivers. Due to lack of equipment, assistive technology, and health care access in many countries, poor nutrition may result, which can hinder normal childhood development. Additionally, difficulty with positioning, and inadequate head support may hamper feeding and eating for young children. Dr. Rabaey supervised graduate students in a mixed-methods research project in Uganda to assess the impact of the chair she is co-developing with Spoon Foundation. Pilot research results indicated an improvement of responsive feeding behaviors, including increased eye contact between caregiver and child, increases in the child's ability to anticipate the spoon and cup, increased positive interaction between the caregiver and child, increased time available between bites of food, and increased positive facial responses from the child (Bruno, 2022). Parents also reported improved ease and enjoyment of feeding their child. One parent remarked "Previous feeding, the baby was passive, like it was forceful feeding because of how they hold her or the posture. But now when she's seated comfortable in the chair, [I] feel it can even make [me] want to feed." Another parent commented, "It helps [me] to be able to feed the baby well, in terms of sitting." Overall, both qualitative and quantitative data revealed the benefit of the chair.

Projects such as this exemplify work aimed at improving conditions that promote participation through improved access to resources and strategies to enhance occupational engagement. When access to resources and services previously unavailable benefit families, the principles and outcomes of occupational justice are addressed.

Occupational Injustice and Deprivation

Earlier in the chapter, five forms of occupational injustice were identified (**occupational apartheid, occupational deprivation, occupational alienation, occupational marginalization,** and **occupational imbalance**). This section will cover one of the earlier types of **occupational justice** identified in the literature, that of occupational deprivation. Specific examples will be discussed along with suggestions for occupational therapists.

Occupational deprivation refers to a restriction in the ability to participate in occupations for reasons outside of the individual's control. Such restrictions may occur due to personal (e.g., health reasons) or structural/societal reasons such as institutionalization, incarceration, displacement, political reasons, and geographic locale. Similar to many of the other concepts discussed in this book, occupational deprivation may affect individuals, groups, and populations.

Chapter 5 discussed sociocultural influences on occupation. Our occupational choices and patterns are influenced by our cultural norms, beliefs, and values. Yet many experience barriers, either temporarily or long term, to occupational participation. Consider the populations hard hit by hurricanes, earthquakes, or flooding. The loss of home, livelihood, and geographical places of safety are not only disrupted, they may cause long-term occupational deprivation. Whiteford (2010) distinguished occupational deprivation from **occupational disruption**, suggesting that occupational deprivation is a "state of prolonged preclusion from engagement in occupations of necessity and/or meaning due to factors which stand outside of the control of the individual" (p. 201), whereas occupational disruption is marked by a temporary or transient change in occupational engagement, which is sometimes under the control of the individual (e.g., a move). For instance, if someone contracts a temporary illness such as a respiratory condition, the person is often able to return to meaningful occupations after healing from a mild sickness; this would be considered occupational disruption. Conversely, a refugee displaced by war will often experience occupational deprivation over time. The situation of being displaced from one's home, often with few resources, and settling in a new land, not only disrupts the occupations of the refugees, it may cause extended occupational deprivation.

The concepts of occupational disruption and occupational deprivation may have some overlap, as in recent years, conditions such as the Covid-19 pandemic not only caused temporary occupational disruption for many with the acute onset of illness, but those who are experiencing long Covid have prolonged occupational deprivation, some not ever having the ability to return to work or have the same level of occupational engagement. Whiteford asserted that the major difference between occupational deprivation and disruption is that occupational disruption is temporary and with the appropriate supportive conditions may be resolved. The following are examples of structural influences that may cause occupational deprivation.

Social Determinants of Health

Social determinants of health (SDOH), introduced earlier in this book include (a) economic stability, (b) education access and quality, (c) health care access and quality, (d) the neighborhood and built environment, and (e) the social and community context (Office of Disease Prevention and Promotion, 2022). Disparities within each of these categories may contribute to occupational deprivation. For example, an individual in substandard housing living in poverty and working three jobs has limited opportunity for occupational balance, and time to engage in health promoting activities. Additionally, those without health insurance or access to health care services lack the preventative health care needed. For instance, in the United States during the pandemic, BIPOC (Black,

Table 6.1 Occupational deprivation and social determinants of health

Occupational deprivation (example)	Social determinants of health
Client with quadriplegia who has limited access to the community	Social and community context
Poor rural youth with low access to meaningful occupation, thus leading to substance abuse	Neighborhood and built environment Economic stability Social and community context Neighborhood and built environment
Children who must take the bus one hour each way to school, thus limiting their ability to complete homework and participate in leisure at home	Neighborhood and built environment Social and community context Education access and quality
Individual in a geographic area with limited access to vaccines, thus contracting serious Covid-19, followed by long Covid, limiting energy for occupational participation	Health care access and quality Social and community context Neighborhood and built environment
Individual incarcerated for several years	Social and community context

Adapted from Reitz and Graham (2019), p. 678.

Indigenous, People of Color) individuals and those in marginalized communities not only had less access to the vaccine, due to the disparities they had higher rates of infection and more serious complications and long-term effects as well (Andraska et al., 2021). Such disparities can lead to occupational deprivation through loss of meaningful work, decreased access to healthy occupations, and loss of ability to partake in daily occupations.

Occupational therapists may use techniques to understand the impact of social determinants on an individual's life and occupational participation. Reitz and Graham (2019) stressed the importance of occupational therapy practitioners considering social determinants of health and their impact on occupational engagement. The authors suggested that questions within the occupational profile may ask what specifically keeps clients from participating in favorite activities. Additional questions may consider the connection of social determinants of health with occupational engagement and ways to facilitate increased participation along with working through the societal barriers to participation. Table 6.1 provides examples of the connection between social determinants of health and occupational deprivation.

Work/Employment/Unemployment

Within industrialized societies, work is often equated with personal identity, self-esteem and self-worth. People are often asked what they do, or what their job is, as if there is an expectation someone works. Although present-day work may look somewhat different than it did prior to the pandemic (e.g., more individuals working online or remotely), it is still an integral part of individual lives and the economic function of society.

Work conditions, unemployment, underemployment, and even overemployment (e.g., having to work excessive hours to meet financial needs) can all be a source of occupational deprivation. Within many societies, work takes up a third or more of the day and, depending on the satisfaction with work, provides occupational engagement and may have additional benefits such as cognitive, physical, and social opportunities. The loss of work (either voluntarily or involuntarily) may contribute to occupational deprivation. Such loss not only includes total loss of work, but involuntary part-time work caused by down-sizing and the loss of hours, which may affect an individual's benefits, financial status, and life satisfaction. Involuntary part-time work is often found in higher numbers in marginalized populations and contributes to poverty wages that may affect personal well-being, health, and other SDH (Blake et al., 2019).

Client, geographical, and societal factors influence access to meaningful productive work. For instance, there are often barriers to persons with disabilities finding, securing, and keeping a job. Jakobsen (2004) conducted a qualitative study that suggested that persons with disabilities often have difficulty finding positions that match their abilities and that often workplaces are not prepared or fully open to employing persons with disabilities. This may further cause occupational deprivation and alienation, particularly when lack of livable wages interferes with ability to engage in desired daily activities such as leisure opportunities or going out with friends. Such disparities are often magnified in low- and middle-income countries due to varying views of disability, limited resources, and lack of infrastructure for sustainable programs and supports related to employment for persons with disabilities, thus affecting rate of employment (Morwane et al., 2021).

Strategies for intervention cited in the literature to address occupational deprivation and detrimental effects of unemployment or underemployment include addressing underlying personal and contextual factors causing the employment conditions, working to change systematic and political structures affecting poor employment conditions, and consideration of mediating factors that may help decrease the ill effects of unemployment or underemployment; these include the provisions of resources, consideration of volunteer work when appropriate, and consideration of leisure supports that enhance life satisfaction (Blake et al., 2019; Morwane et al., 2021; Whiteford, 2010).

Institutionalization

Within sociology and mental health, the term **institutionalization** is often used to denote long-term residence in a jail, prison, or psychiatric institution. There are personal and sociological effects of prolonged institutional residence, which may include limited opportunity for occupational engagement and difficulty leaving the institution (e.g., following a long prison term or hospitalization). Historically, institutionalization in asylums, paired with institutional neglect, often left individuals without basic necessities, human rights, and opportunities for meaningful activities. Although efforts have been made to increase meaningful activity, treatment, and personal goal attainment in many institutions (e.g., long-term mental health programs), there are continued concerns with lack of funding, minimal occupational opportunities, and involuntary treatment in many of these facilities (Warburton & Stahl, 2020). This lack of access to meaningful activities has lasting physical and psychological effects. For instance, youth who grow up in institutionalized settings may experience higher levels of psychopathology and difficulties with cognition (Tibu et al., 2016), which may subsequently affect occupational participation. Additional concerns arise in settings with incarcerated populations.

Concerns related to occupational deprivation because of institutionalization are magnified for those in jails (shorter term) and prisons (longer term). Globally, there is an over-representation of racial/ethnic minorities and socially disadvantaged individuals in the prison system, particularly in the United States (Munoz, 2019). Further, a significant number of individuals in these systems have major mental health conditions, many of which are not addressed or are under-addressed in the prison system. Within the prison system, occupational deprivation may occur, with limited opportunity for meaningful activity and poor access to educational opportunities (Davis et al., 2013). Thus, once an individual is discharged after prolonged incarceration, opportunities may be limited and skills lacking to assimilate back into society. Prisons are often in highly secure fairly remote areas and impose restrictions on occupational engagement (Whiteford, 2010). Rationale for such restrictions may include the safety of the prisoners and guards (e.g., preventing access to sharps), or lack of resources to provide adequate opportunities for meaningful occupations. Thus, the routines may become rote without novelty, and prisoners may suffer from boredom, influencing the desire to seek opportunities for engagement. Such boredom and lack of engagement may compound psychological stress and have other detrimental health effects.

Munoz (2019) stated that criminal justice systems often create barriers to providing occupation-based practice, given that their primary goal is security rather than rehabilitation. Within this environment clients may become deprived of social, leisure, and work opportunities such that reintegration may be difficult because they may lack the skills for re-entry into society. Although occupational therapy is often absent in these settings, when available, goals may include skill development, and strategies for community reintegration and relapse prevention.

Displacement

Issues such as wars, refugeeism, and natural disaster cause not only disruption in daily life and occupational patterns, but also long-term deprivation, particularly in instances involving loss of home, and in some cases the need to leave the geographical locale in which one lives. In many instances, displacement involving mass migration also affects not only the migrants, but also the receiving communities, given the need to find resources and housing for populations entering the area. It is important to note that there are differences in, for instance, immigrants, who choose to move to a new locale or country, and refugees or asylum seekers, who are compelled to leave due to political unrest, war, or some other reason. In addition, displacement may occur internally (within the same country), or externally (to a new country). The United States continues to be the country receiving the highest number of people in resettlement (Solf & Rehberg, 2021), yet often resources are lacking, political opinions interfere with efforts, and the voice of the refugee or immigrant is not always heard. Such displacement results in occupational deprivation, takes an emotional and physical toll and affects individuals, families, and populations. Globally, resettlement of refugees, immigrants, and asylum seekers brings social exclusion and lack of opportunities for education, work, and integration into society (Mirza, 2012; Phillimore & Goodson, 2006).

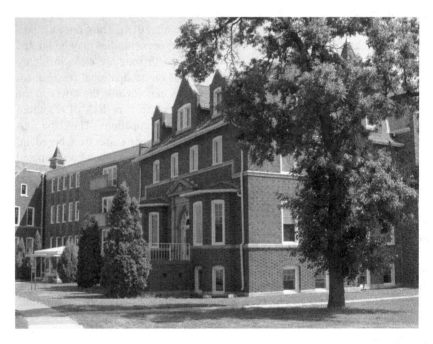

Figure 6.2 Institutionalization may cause occupational deprivation (photo courtesy of Kristine Haertl)

Resettlement often involves three phases: identification, access, and submission of the case (Solf & Rehberg, 2021) The office of the United Nations High Commissioner for Refugees (UNHCR) initially *identifies* categories of refugees' need for resettlement and potential receiving countries; the second phase, *access*, involves the receiving country gathering information; and the final phase, *submission of the case*, includes eligibility for immigrant or refugee status. Within the process, challenges may include bureaucratic red tape, long waits, differing political ideologies toward immigrants, and strained resources.

In addition to the stress placed on immigrants and refugees in the moving process, often there is a history of trauma that must be addressed, given that situations influencing migration often involve war, abuse, political unrest, and lack of adequate basic needs. Initial resettlement may include massive camps, temporary housing, and conditions that lack rich occupational opportunity. If populations have traveled hundreds of miles, they have likely had inadequate resources for food, clothing, and necessary self-care. This may be compounded by poor health and malnourishment, all of which contribute to deprived conditions. Additional barriers after resettlement may include language differences, adjustment to new cultures, and adaptation to new geographic locations and climates. Yet it is important to note that refugees and immigrants may also see the new locale as a place of opportunity and potential growth.

Implications for Occupational Therapy

Bailliard et al. (2020) wrote that occupational therapy has roots in justice efforts, noting that its founders in 1917 included social activists who advocated for the "occupational" rights of marginalized populations. Occupational therapists often work with many displaced populations in a variety of settings, including the health care and social systems. Therapists assist these clients to facilitate adjustment to their new settings, addressing self-care, life skills, leisure, work, and other relevant occupational areas. According to the World Federation of Occupational Therapists (2019), it is of high importance that therapists are client-centered, respectful, and sensitive to the cultural traditions of these clients.

As noted in Chapter 5, occupational therapists may apply justice principles at the micro (client/individual), meso (organizational), or macro (societal) level. At the micro or client level, a therapist collaborates with the individual to understand their *narrative* (personal story), personal values, and life goals, which, according to Bailliard and Aldrich (2017) is closely tied to issues of justice. At this level therapists can better identify and realize their influence within the health care system, appreciating the structures that can unjustly disadvantage a client's opportunities to engage in meaningful occupations such as paid work, parental caregiving, and leisure (e.g., is the client homeless, does the client have access to transportation, food, living resources and vocational opportunities?). Intervention strategies thus draw from the client's narratives and goals, seeking to identify strategies that address any occupational injustices that may occur. For instance, if a 46-year-old client with schizophrenia loves to color yet is in a system that doesn't consider coloring "age appropriate," the therapist needs to acknowledge personal and cultural differences in working with the client and find ways to encourage the client's occupational interests and engagement. Intervention at the meso (organizational) level, seeks to address occupational justice through cultural awareness, education, and change. For example, with the occupation of toileting and using the bathroom, personal access due to disability status or gender identity may restrict use. Assuring access through universal design such as international symbols (and/or bilingual signage) for public restrooms would be an example of addressing occupational justice at a systems level. Addressing individual and systems biases and structural injustice seeks to change the underlying structural issues that limit participation.

Finally, at the macro level, therapists can use frameworks such as the Participatory Occupational Justice Framework (Whiteford et al., 2017) discussed earlier, to develop community partnerships and promote lasting social change that encourages access to participation. For instance, recently in a Midwestern state in the United States, therapists, students, teachers, and staff educated the public and raised money to fund an accessible playground to assure access by all students seeking to participate in recess and outdoor play activities.

While productivity standards and institutional expectations may make it difficult for occupational therapists to spend extensive time advocating for occupational justice efforts, Bailliard et al. (2020) noted that therapists can still affect change through their collaboration with individuals, communities, and populations. The reader may wish to review Box 6.1, presented earlier, as another useful example of an occupational therapist using occupational justice principles.

Summary

This chapter has presented definitions, terms, and frameworks of occupational justice. Key terms within occupational justice include occupational rights, occupational apartheid, occupational deprivation, occupational imbalance, occupational alienation, and occupational marginalization. These injustices often overlap and affect individuals and communities. Occupational therapists may work at the individual, system, and population level to promote occupational justice through applying the frameworks outlined in the chapter. One type of occupational justice, occupational deprivation, was presented along with conditions that may cause deprivation in relation to social determinants of health, employment/unemployment, institutionalization, and displacement. Recognizing injustice and addressing it at the individual and collective level is essential to the health and well-being of communities.

BOX 6.2 THE POINT IS:

- Occupational justice refers to equal opportunity for engagement in meaningful occupations.
- Major terms associated with occupational injustice include occupational apartheid, occupational deprivation, occupational marginalization, occupational alienation, and occupational imbalance. Each of these may indicate a violation of occupational rights.
- Conditions that may case occupational deprivation include underemployment and unemployment, institutionalization, and displacement.
- Therapists may apply the Participatory Occupational Justice Framework (POJF) at the individual, systems, or population level to work toward occupational justice.

Acknowledgement

The authors thank Paula Rabaey, PhD, MPH, OTR/L for kindly sharing details and photos regarding her work in Zambia.

References

Andraska, E. A., Alabi, O., Dorsey, C., Erben, Y., Velazquez, G., Franco-Mesa, C., & Sachdev, U. (2021). Healthcare disparities during the Covid-19 pandemic. *Seminars in Vascular Surgery*, *34*(3), 82–88. https://doi.org/10.1053/j.semvascsurg.2021.08 .002

Bailliard A., & Aldrich R. (2017). Occupational justice in everyday occupational therapy practice. In N. Pollard & D. Sakellariou (Eds.), *Occupational therapies without borders: Integrating justice with practice* (2nd ed., pp. 83–94). Elsevier.

Bailliard, A. L., Dallman, A. R., Carroll, A., Lee, B. D., Szendrey S. (2020). Doing occupational justice: A central dimension of everyday occupational therapy practice. *Canadian Journal of Occupational Therapy*, *87*(2), 144–152. https://doi.org /10.1177/0008417419898930

Blake, B. A., Kim, T., Liu, T. Y., & Deemer, D. E. (2019). Moderators of involuntary part time work and life satisfaction: A latent deprivation approach. *Professional Psychology Research and Practice*, *51*(3), 257–267. https://doi.org/10.1037/ pro0000268

Bruno, N. (2022). *The influence of the Spoon feeding chair on the caregiver dyad.* Master's Thesis. https://sophia.stkate.edu/ma_osot/33/

Canadian Association of Occupational Therapists (2022). *Canadian Occupational Performance Measure.* Author. www.thecopm.ca

Davis, L. M., Bozick, R., Steele, J. L., Saunders, J., & Miles, J. (2013). *Evaluating the effectiveness of correctional education: A meta-analysis of programs that provide education to incarcerated adults*. Rand Corporation and the Bureau of Justice Assistance.

Durocher, E., Gibson, B. E., & Rappolt, S. (2014). Occupational justice: A conceptual review. *Journal of Occupational Science, 21*(4), 418–438. www.tandfonline.com/doi /full/10.1080/14427591.2013.775692

Hammell, K. W. (2008). Reflections on ... well-being and occupational rights. *Canadian Journal of Occupational Therapy, 75*(1), 61–64. https://doi.org/10.2182/cjot.07.007

Jakobsen, K. (2004) If work doesn't work: How to enable occupational justice. *Journal of Occupational Science, 11*(3), 125–134. https://doi.org/10.1080/14427591.2004 .9686540

Kronenberg, F., & Pollard, N. (2005). Overcoming occupational apartheid: A preliminary exploration of the political nature of occupational therapy. In F. Kronenberg, S. S. Algado, & N. Pollard (Eds.), *Occupational therapy without borders: Learning from the spirit of survivors* (pp. 58–86). Elsevier Churchill Livingstone Migration Policy Institute: The resettlement gap: A record number of global refugees, but few are resettled. www.migrationpolicy.org/article/refugee-resettlement-gap

Mirza, M. (2012). Occupational upheaval during resettlement and migration: Findings of a global ethnography with refugees with disabilities. *OTJR: Occupation, Participation and Health, 1*, S6–S14. https://doi.org/10.3928/15394492-20110906 -04

Morwane, R. E., Dada, S., & Bornman, J. (2021). Barriers to and facilitators of employment of persons with disabilities in low- and middle-income countries: A scoping review. *African Journal of Disability, 10*, a33. https://doi.org/10.4102/ajod.v10i0.833

Munoz, J. P. (2019). Mental health practice in criminal justice systems. In C. Brown, V. C. Stoffel, & J. P. Munoz (Eds.), *Occupational therapy in mental health: A vision for participation* (2nd ed., pp. 615–641). F. A. Davis.

Office of Disease Prevention and Promotion. (2022). *Healthy people 2030: Social determinants of health*. https://health.gov/healthypeople/priority-areas/social -determinants-health

Phillimore, J., & Goodson, L. (2006). Problem or opportunity? Asylum seekers, refugees, employment, and social exclusion in deprived areas. *Urban Studies, 43*(10), 1715–1736. www.jstor.org/stable/43197399

Reitz, S. M. & Graham, K. (2019). Health promotion theories. In B. A. Schell & G. Gillen (Eds.), *Willard and Spackman's occupational therapy* (13th ed., pp. 675–692). Lippincott Williams & Wilkins.

Stadnyk, R., Townsend, E., & Wilcock, A. (2010). Occupational justice. In C. H. Christiansen & E. A. Townsend (Eds.), *Introduction to occupation: The art and science of living* (2nd ed., pp. 329–358). Pearson Education.

Solf, B., & Rehberg, K. (2021). *The resettlement gap: A record number of global refugees but few are resettled*. Migration Policy Institute. www.migrationpolicy.org/article /refugee-resettlement-gap#:~:text=Historically%2C%20the%20United%20States %20has,per%20capita%20rate%20of%20resettlement

Tibu, F., Sheridan, M. A., McLaughlin, K. A., Nelson, C. A., Fox, N. A., & Zeanah, C. H. (2016). Disruptions of working memory and inhibition mediate the association between exposure to institutionalization and symptoms of attention deficit hyperactivity disorder. *Psychological Medicine, 46*(3), 529–541. https://doi.org/10 .1017/S0033291715002020

Townsend, E. A., & Whiteford, G. (2005). A participatory occupational justice framework: Population-based processes of practice. In F. Kronenberg, S. Simó Algado, & N. Pollard (Eds.), *Occupational therapy without borders: Learning from the spirit of survivors* (pp. 110–126). Elsevier.

Townsend, E. A. & Wilcock, A. A. (2004). Occupational justice and client-centred practice: A dialogue in progress. *Canadian Journal of Occupational Therapy, 71*(2), 75–87. https://doi.org/10.1177/000841740407100203

Warburton, K., & Stahl, S. M. (2020). Balancing the pendulum: Rethinking the role of institutionalization in serious mental illness. *CNS Spectrums, 25*(2), 115–118. https:// doi.org/10.1017/S1092852920000176

Whiteford, G. (2000). Occupational deprivation: Global challenge in the new millennium. *British Journal of Occupational Therapy, 63*(5), 200–204. https://doi.org/10.1177 /030802260006300503

Whiteford, G. (2010). Occupational deprivation: Understanding limited participation. In C. H. Christiansen & E. A. Townsend (Eds.), *Introduction to occupation: The art and science of living* (2nd ed., pp. 303–328). Pearson Education.

Whiteford, G., Jones, K., Rahal, C., & Suleman, A. (2018). The Participatory Occupational Justice Framework as a tool for change: Three contrasting case narratives. *Journal of Occupational Science, 25*(4), 497–508. https://doi.org/10.1080/14427591.2018 .1504607

Wilcock, A. A., & Hocking, C. (2015). *An occupational perspective of health* (2nd ed.). Slack.

Wilcock, A. A., & Townsend, E. A. (2000). Occupational justice: Occupational terminology interactive dialogue. *Journal of Occupational Science, 7*(2), 84–86. https://doi.org/10.1080/14427591.2000.9686470

Wilcock, A. A., & Townsend, E. A. (2019). Occupational justice. In B. A. Schell & G. Gillen (Eds.), *Willard and Spackman's occupational therapy* (13th ed., pp. 643–659). Lippincott Williams & Wilkins.

World Federation of Occupational Therapists (2019). *Resource manual: Occupational therapy for displaced persons.* www.wfot.org/resources/wfot-resource-manual -occupational-therapy-for-displaced-persons

Chapter 7

Occupation-based Theories and Practice Models

Introduction

Guiding concepts and frameworks are integral to the practice of a profession. As previously emphasized, the importance of meaningful doing, or occupation, has been a core distinguishing feature of occupational therapy since its inception. The study of occupation and foundations of occupational science are key to theories, models, and frames of reference that guide practice. As described in Chapter 1, definitions of the term occupation have varied through the years, and the *doing* of daily activities is typically a central feature of these definitions, along with the meaning or perceived value of an activity. This chapter extends that discussion, illustrating how ideas about occupation have evolved as theories and practice models have developed over time.

McColl (2015) identified occupation as "purposeful or meaningful activities in which humans engage as part of their normal daily lives" (p. 53). Schell et al. (2014) extended this further to describe occupations as "the things people do that occupy their time and attention; meaningful purposeful activity; the personal activities that individuals choose or need to engage in and the ways in which each individual actually experiences them" (p. 1237). The Occupational Therapy Practice Framework, 4th edition (American Occupational Therapy Association, 2020, p. 79), defines occupation as

> Everyday personalized activities that people do as individuals, in families, and with communities to occupy time and bring meaning and purpose to life. Occupations can involve the execution of multiple activities for completion and can result in various outcomes. The broad range of occupations is categorized as activities of daily living, instrumental activities of daily living, health management, rest and sleep, education, work, play, leisure, and social participation.

Yet some authors question specific categorizations of occupation and assert the importance of cultural considerations and context within the meaning of

DOI: 10.4324/9781003242185-7

occupation (Cutchin, 2004; Reed et al., 2011; Robinson Johnson & Dickie, 2019). Despite differing but related definitions, common to the definitions and features of occupation-based practice are *doing, purpose,* and *meaning*; recognizing that the context in which activities occur also influences these elements.

These evolving ideas about occupation have influenced the development of frameworks, or models, to guide thinking about research and practice in occupational therapy. Conceptual model development in occupational therapy began in the 1950s, blossomed in the 1980s, and has continued, with more recent emphasis on critiquing, refining, and validating existing models rather than on the creation of original new models. Common to these models are symbolic depictions of the relationships of key components, and almost universally these include the individual *person,* the context including situational and *environmental factors,* and the *occupation* (Reid et al., 2019).

Models also address how the occupation is completed, often termed as the **occupational performance**. The level or quality of performance depends on the goodness of fit between the person, occupation, and contextual factors (Brown, 2019). Within occupational therapy, the use of occupation has been described as both a means, using occupation in the therapeutic process of doing, and an end— the desired occupational goal of therapy (Gray, 1998). Occupation-based models help us conceptualize the interaction of the person, environment, and occupation and identify strategies to approach the occupational therapy process to maximize occupational performance. Each model is unique in helping us understand engagement in occupation.

This chapter is intended to provide a brief overview of some commonly used occupation-based theories and **practice models**. Textbooks differ in their definitions of models and frames of reference. Thus, for the purpose of this chapter, five commonly cited frameworks are presented as representative occupation-based models of practice. This chapter is not meant to be an exhaustive survey of existing models, but rather to present a sample of widely used occupation-based models to provide readers with an overview of their key concepts and how those concepts are applied. The intent is to show how the **clinical reasoning** process may be guided by the different models as practitioners use them for assessment and intervention.

Before the models are summarized, it may be worthwhile to consider the notion of **eclecticism**, which can be defined simply as the process of deriving ideas from many different sources. In occupational therapy practice, practitioners sometimes claim to be eclectic, or to draw their guidance from many practice models. At first glance, this seems reasonable. One might ask: "Why not choose the best ideas from each model?" The answer is that there is nothing *inherently* wrong with eclecticism as long as a practitioner has a clear understanding of how a given concept from one model fits appropriately within the context of another. But this is more difficult than it seems because a thorough understanding of the frameworks and components of different models *based on their use in practice* is generally needed to do this expertly.

Occupational therapy practitioners are thus wise to recognize that established models of practice have evolved over time, been subjected to analysis and study, and refined. As a result, they tend to have internal consistency, meaning that their descriptions and definitions, assessments, intervention strategies, and reporting methods are designed to work together. Thus, a thorough understanding of the frameworks used to guide the occupational therapy process is imperative. All professionals have an ethical responsibility to select, apply, and be educated on the best or most appropriate approach for each individual client from among those that are feasible (Rogers, 1983).

Person–Environment–Occupation–Performance (PEOP) Model

The Person–Environment–Occupation–Performance model (PEOP) is a top-down client-centered approach, originally developed in 1988, that emphasizes the interdependence of person factors, environmental factors, and occupation on occupational performance (Christiansen & Baum, 1991; Christiansen et al., 2015). This model is a social ecological model, in that it considers a broad range of factors to guide the occupational therapy practitioner in identifying the client's strengths and areas of need in conjunction with environmental factors (current living circumstances, access to resources, social connections, etc.) in the client's life that affect occupational performance.

The model identifies three domains viewed as integral to occupational therapy practice, *person factors* (cognition, psychological, physiological, sensory, motor, and spiritual), *environmental factors* (culture, social determinants, social support and capital, education and policy, physical and natural and assistive technology), and *occupations* (activities, tasks, and roles) the person wants and needs to do in their daily lives (Baum et al., 2015). As depicted in Figure 7.1, the doing of the activity is influenced by the environment and person factors, which subsequently affects occupational performance. Therapeutic outcomes of PEOP strive to support occupational role performance, identity, life satisfaction, health, and optimal function (Bass et al., 2015). More recent versions of the model also emphasize the narrative, which considers the client's background and personal characteristics in order to guide occupational therapy goals and intervention approaches. In addition to focusing on the individual person, newer versions of the model have added populations and organizations that acknowledge current paradigms of occupational therapy in global health (Cole & Tufano, 2020).

PEOP in Practice

The use of PEOP in the occupational therapy process includes four components, (a) the narrative, (b) assessment and evaluation, (c) intervention, and (d) outcome phases (Bass et al., 2015). The *narrative phase* includes gathering information

The Person Environment Occupation Performance (PEOP) Model

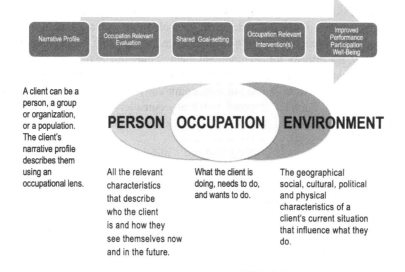

Figure 7.1 PEOP model (based on PEOP model, Baum et al., 2015, revised by Christiansen, 2023)

on the client's past and current perceptions of strengths and difficulties in occupational performance. Consideration must also be given to personal meaning, choice, attitude, and motivation as these influence goal setting in a collaborative client–therapist approach. The *assessment and evaluation phase* uses evidence-based assessments to determine constraints/barriers and strengths/enablers to meaningful occupational engagement. Assessments are selected to address the person, occupation, and environment and may pertain to any occupational area including ADL, IADL, rest/sleep, education, work, play/leisure, and social participation. Although the model has not adopted specific assessment tools, Cole and Tufano (2020) asserted that within this model a wide range of instruments may be used, such as interest and role checklists, the Canadian Occupational Performance Measure (COPM) (Law et al., 2014), and the Activity Card Sort (Baum & Edwards, 2008). Additional tools may be selected that fit the model if they consider the core occupational areas and the interaction of client, environment, and occupational performance.

The *intervention phase* of the model emphasizes a client-centered approach to developing an action plan to address goal areas based on the strengths and needs/barriers identified in the *assessment/evaluation phase*. Interventions used within the model consider the goodness of fit between the client and environment and the modalities needed to maximize occupational performance in prioritized areas. Consideration of a client's priorities based on importance and value is necessary, since the client may have difficulty with multiple occupations.

For instance, even though Clark, an 18-year-old male with a C5 quadriplegia from a recent accident has difficulty with independent dressing, which takes him over an hour, his priority for occupational therapy may not be to work on dressing but on the ability to independently use transportation to attend his local university. Thus, the focus of therapy may be community mobility skills rather than personal dressing. Such an approach to therapy considers the client's priorities and values, while also considering the environment and subsequent occupational performance.

The last and final *outcome phase* includes a discussion between the therapist and client related to desired outcomes of proposed interventions. This phase goes beyond consideration of the individual client's goals to include outcomes that affect the organizations, groups, and individuals with whom the client interacts. According to Bass et al. (2015), this broader view of outcomes helps establish the value of occupational therapy beyond the client, and to reflect how individuals as well as groups and populations benefit. This illustrates a systems approach that more fully accounts for the transactional nature of the person, environment, and occupation and how the components of the model interrelate. Every change has the potential to affect the entire system.

Person–Environment–Occupation (PEO) Model

Similar to the PEOP, the Person–Environment–Occupation (PEO) model emphasizes the transactional relationship of the *person*, the *environment*, and the *occupations* performed. This model was conceptualized by Canadian scholars and clinicians as a framework for occupational therapists to understand occupational performance (Law et al., 1996). The model's client-centered approach embraces autonomy, diversity, empowerment, the therapeutic partnership, contextual congruence (the environmental fit with the occupation), and flexibility (Cole & Tufano, 2020). The PEO model emphasizes the relationship of the person performing an occupation in various environments through time (Strong & Reberio-Gruhl, 2019). Change within one element (e.g., the environment) affects the other components. For instance, an individual with cognition and mobility challenges may have high levels of functional mobility in a one-level accessible home, but if the environment is changed to a multi-level large building with low accessibility, the occupational performance is affected.

The conceptualization of *person* in PEO acknowledges not only the affective (feeling), cognitive (thinking), and doing (physical) elements of the individual, but also the spiritual realm, an element that is seen as integral to giving meaning to the occupations. The categories identified in the *environment* component of the model include cultural, institutional, physical, and social elements of the environment. For instance, cultural environments would include ethnic, political, religious, and other environments that affect the cultural context. Examples of physical environments may include a classroom, workplace, living area, or city park and countryside. Institutional elements may involve the political systems, legislative bodies, and institutional rules that may affect the occupational performance. Finally, the social elements involve the relationships, social support, and social elements. The *occupation* in this model typically refers to the Canadian occupational therapy classifications, including self-care, productivity, and leisure. Yet, as mentioned earlier in the chapter, some have criticized this conceptualization as too narrow and representative of Caucasian, Eurocentric North American values. Levels of occupation within the model may be understood as the activity (basic unit of the task), task (smallest component of an occupation), and the occupation (set of tasks) (Baptiste, 2018; Cole & Tufano, 2020). The concept of **occupational load** has also recently been added to refer "to not only the physical aspects of a work activity but also the number of different roles, tasks and occupations that a person wants, needs, or is expected to do" (Cole & Tufano, 2020, p. 171). Consideration of occupational load is integral to prioritizing goals and interventions for therapy.

PEO in Practice

Evaluation and intervention in the PEO model take into account the interactions of each of the elements of the model. The person–occupation (P x O) relationship considers the individual and occupation. For example, Shayna, a 78-year-old female with a recent right CVA (stroke in the right hemisphere) would like to return to cooking. Additional considerations include the fact that she is highly familiar with cooking and is regaining strength in her left arm. The occupation–environment (O x E) combination acknowledges the importance of the environmental impact on the occupation. In the example provided above, the arrangement of Shayna's kitchen will affect her ability to resume cooking. The person–environment (P x E) also considers the individual in the environment. Shayna is familiar with her kitchen and has access to home health rehabilitation providers, which may further support her return to a valued occupation (cooking).

The PEO evaluation process uses all components and relationships in the model, identifies priority occupational performance areas, and formulates a plan based on the analysis described above. Assessment tools such as the Canadian Occupational Performance Measure (Law et al., 2014) further identify the client's priorities in the occupational therapy process. Intervention within the model emphasizes the collaborative partnership and therapeutic use of self to empower the client toward improved occupational performance. Focus is on

occupational enablement that examines intervention solutions to promote occupational performance.

Canadian Model of Occupational Performance and Engagement (CMOP-E)

The Canadian Model of Occupational Performance and Engagement (CMOP-E) evolved from the Canadian Model of Occupational Performance, which was created and adopted by the Canadian Association of Occupational Therapists in 1997. Similar to the PEO and PEOP models, the *person*, *occupation*, and *environment* are the main components in the model. Key concepts that have been central to the Canadian approach to occupational therapy include (a) occupation as the core of occupational therapy, (b) spirituality as the central core of the person, (c) the experiential nature of occupation, (d) a client-centered focus, (e) the environment as influential on occupational performance, and (f) enablement as a core concept of occupational therapy (Law & Laver-Fawcett, 2013; Townsend & Polatajko, 2007, 2013). Recent versions of the model emphasize the role of the occupational therapist in using knowledge and skills (including client relationship skills, known as therapeutic use of self) to enable occupation. The idea of enablement was added to the model to emphasize important factors beyond successful performance of the occupation to include engagement, or the active involvement of the person in the occupation (McColl et al., 2015). Skills used by the therapist within the therapy process to enable occupation include adapting, advocating, coaching, collaborating, designing, educating, building, engaging, and specializing (McColl et al., 2015).

CMOP-E in Practice

As previously discussed, the interrelated nature of the person, environment, and occupation means that a change in one component will affect the relationship of all dimensions of the model and may facilitate or disrupt occupational performance. A core assessment tool in this model, the Canadian Occupational Performance Measure (Law et al., 1990, 2014) was developed through a collaborative effort between Health and Welfare Canada and the Canadian Association of Occupational Therapists. The tool has informed the development of the Canadian occupation-based models and provides a semi-structured interview that explores the client's perspectives and priorities in areas of self-care, productivity, and leisure. Clients rate their top five difficulties in performance and the level of satisfaction in occupational therapy in order to develop goals for therapy. Client factors such as cognition and insight should be considered and therapists may partner this evaluation with a functional occupation-based assessment that involves actual performance.

Important concepts for intervention in this model along with the PEO model are identified by Cole and Tufano (2020) as follows:

- Presence of an occupational challenge
- Need for occupational enablement (considerations of solutions to enable occupational performance)
- Client-specific goals, challenges, and solutions considering the client's occupations, roles, patterns, and goals
- A multidisciplinary knowledge base (embracing the complexity of occupations)
- Reasoning that deals with complexity (a therapist's knowledge of the transactional relationship of PEO and the therapeutic use of self).

Emphasis is placed throughout the occupational therapy process on the clinical reasoning and therapeutic skills of the occupational therapist in using a client-centered approach to enable occupational performance.

Occupational Adaptation

The **occupational adaptation** model (Schkade & Schultz, 1992a, 1992b), emphasizes occupation as a means through which humans adapt to develop mastery. Three key components of this model include the *person*, the *occupational environment*, and the *interaction* between the person and occupational environment (Schkade & Shultz, 1992a). Based on general systems theory, the model asserts that the person receives feedback from the environment, occupation, and outcome of the interaction and thus adapts. The concept of an occupational challenge leads the individual through a *press* towards mastery. Within the model, "*occupations* are activities characterized by three properties: (1) active participation, (2) meaning to the person, and (3) a product that is the output of a process" (Schkade & Schultz, 1992a, p. 831). The model identifies *adaptation* as the process that occurs via a change in the functional status of the individual in that person's movement toward mastery over the occupational challenge. Finally, the client's state of **competency** in occupational functioning (being able to do what they are currently unable to do) is referred to as *occupational adaptation*. The model asserts that adaptation occurs through (a), practicing or learning skills from the occupation, (b) modifying the occupation, and (c) learning a new occupation. Thus, occupational adaptation is a culmination of the interactive process of the person with the environment and the internal adaptive process that occurs through occupational engagement (Schultz, 2014). Additional key concepts include that occupations (a) actively involve the person, (b) hold meaning for the person, and (c) involve either a process or product (Cole & Tufano, 2020). Key assumptions identified in the model are as follows:

- Occupations provide natural developmental opportunities for adaptation.
- Occupational roles include demands and expectations for performance (including context considerations).
- When an individual is unable to meet the demands of the person, task or environment, a disruption in occupational adaptation occurs.
- A person's adaptive capacity is impacted by impairment, physical or emotional disability, and stressful life transitions throughout the lifespan.
- There is a direct correlation of a person's level of dysfunction and the need for change in adaptation; inability to adapt with mastery may lead to poor occupational performance.
- Once an individual's ability to adapt reaches sufficient mastery of self and society they will experience successful occupational performance.

Each of these assumptions is integral to the occupational therapy process in working toward promotion of occupational adaptation and mastery of occupational performance.

Grajo (2019) has reconceptualized the model and asserted that describing occupational adaptation as both a process and product in occupational therapy practice is problematic (Grajo et al., 2018; Grajo, 2019). He proposes that occupational adaptation: a) is a normative internal human process, and b) is an intervention process that may guide an occupational therapist's critical thinking and clinical reasoning both in the therapeutic relationship and process.

Occupational Adaptation in Practice

The focus of intervention in occupational adaptation is directed at improving the client's occupational adaptation process, the natural process that occurs through development (Schkade & Schultz, 1992b). The authors of this model assert that congenital and acquired conditions (e.g., a traumatic brain injury or serious illness) can impair the individual's occupational adaptation process. Therapists direct and affect the client's ability to generate adaptive responses and work toward mastery. This model acknowledges that a client's functional skills are important, but that the main focus of intervention should be on facilitating occupational adaptation. The authors assert that such adaptation benefits current as well as future occupational function (Schkade & Schultz, 1992a, 1992b). Three key subprocesses of adaptation proposed by the authors include (a) the *generation* of the adaptive response, (b) the *evaluation* and self-reflection of how effective the response was, and (c) the *integration* of insights gained.

Within occupational adaptation, the therapeutic relationship is integral. The role of the therapist is to facilitate adaptation, leading to improved occupational performance. The evaluation process often involves observation of an activity of interest. Therapists then observe the client's problem solving when occupational challenges occur and facilitate improved adaptation through the intervention process. The initial evaluation process includes data gathering, planning of the activity observed, and evaluation of the process and intervention outcomes. An instrument that may be used to assess occupational adaptation in this model is the Relative Mastery Measurement Scale (George et al., 2004), a questionnaire designed to assess client perception and satisfaction related to mastery of response to occupational challenge. When used in conjunction with observation, the evaluation process leads to plans for **occupation-based interventions** to enhance mastery and adaptation.

Evaluation and intervention in occupational adaptation is dynamic. The developers of the model asserted that the role of the therapist is to facilitate the client's ability to make adaptations; thus, clients are identified as their own agents of change (Cole & Tufano, 2020). This model does not have specific intervention techniques, but instead, proposes a way to think about the client (Schkade & Schultz, 2003). The client directs the occupational role for the focus of therapy and the assessment process identifies what is facilitating and hindering performance. Intervention focuses on the occupational readiness of the client and the specific occupation of focus.

The Model of Human Occupation (MOHO)

The original developers of the Model of Human Occupation were influenced by occupational behavior, a set of ideas that emphasized the normal developmental continuum of human skills from play to work (Woodside, 1976). The framework was developed by Reilly (1962) and motivated by a concern that occupational therapy's reliance on the medical model was ill-suited, inadequate, and inconsistent with the broader wellness-oriented and more occupation-centered roots of the profession.

Reilly emphasized the concepts of competency, achievement, and role, arguing that humans are motivated by their natural inclination to explore and direct their own actions, which in turn enables competency. She proposed that such competence was the consequence of acquiring and mastering the skills necessary for humans in their everyday societal roles.

Influenced by Reilly's work, Gary Kielhofner and Janice Burke, students of Reilly, presented a holistic client-centered model, the Model of Human Occupation (MOHO) to explain human occupation (Kielhofner & Burke, 1980). Within MOHO, the person is conceptualized through an open system by which occupational behavior is the output. Similar to other models, MOHO emphasizes the human drive toward mastery. The influence of the environment, and contextual aspects such as society and culture are acknowledged within the open system. Kielhofner and colleagues later published the first of many books on the Model of Human Occupation to describe the theory, model, and application to occupational therapy (Kielhofner, 1985). MOHO emphasizes that what an individual does in play, work, and self-care (occupations) is a result of environmental factors, motivation, life patterns, and performance capacity. Through occupational engagement, people shape their identities and reaffirm their sense of selves.

MOHO has four key elements, **volition, habituation, performance capacity**, and **environment** (Taylor, 2017). Components of the person in MOHO include *volition* (how the person chooses what they do), *habituation* (how the act of doing is influenced by patterns and routines), and *performance capacity* (the physical and mental capacities within the lived experience); each of these components interacts to affect occupational choice and performance.

The *environment* within MOHO includes physical and social environments. Physical environments include natural environments and built environments (e.g., roads, stairs, etc.). MOHO asserts that the environment in which we perform occupations may have opportunities, resources, demands, and constraints. These factors interact with the person's interests, values, personal causation, roles, habits, and performance capacities and thus the environmental effect on occupational performance differs for each person.

The Model of Human Occupation (MOHO) in Practice

Occupational therapists use MOHO in a client-centered manner to identify strengths and barriers in occupational performance, identify goals, and work toward improved participation. The main therapeutic purpose of MOHO is to restore occupational identity, promote life satisfaction through occupational engagement, and develop competency that meets social and personal expectations (Cole & Tufano, 2020). The therapist's knowledge of MOHO directs the occupational therapy process from evaluation to goal setting, to intervention, and assessment of outcomes.

Kielhofner and Forsyth (2008) identified the following steps for therapeutic reasoning to guide occupational therapy:

1. Generative questions to guide information gathering (guided by the model and aimed at the person factors—volition, habituation, and performance capacity—along with an understanding of the environment)
2. Gathering information on or with the client (may use a structured and non-structured assessment approach)
3. Creating a conceptualization of the client that includes strengths and challenges (synthesized results of the assessment process designed to understand the client and environment)
4. Identifying goals and plans for client engagement and therapeutic strategies (creating goals with the client; identifying occupational engagement opportunities to create change; developing therapeutic strategies to promote change)
5. Implementing and reviewing therapy

6. Collecting information to assess therapy outcomes.

The initial process of understanding the client may involve both formal and informal processes (e.g., structured and unstructured interviews, observations, chart review, etc.). The University of Illinois, Chicago MOHO Clearinghouse (www.moho.uic.edu) houses a number of assessment tools for persons across the lifespan, based on the MOHO model. The following are a sample of MOHO specific tools; a more comprehensive description is provided in Chapter 8.

• Occupational Performance History Interview (OPHI-II) (Kielhofner et al., 2004)
• Occupational Self-Assessment (OSA version 2), short and long forms (Baron et al., 2006)
• Volitional Questionnaire (de las Heras et al., 2007)
• Model of Human Occupation Screening Tool (MOHOST version 2) (Parkinson et al., 2006).

The above tools use interviews, observations, and self-perception to measure areas such as occupational identity, volition, occupational behavior, and occupational performance. Results of the MOHO assessments are used in the occupational therapy process to assess strengths and needs, identify goals, and work to improve occupational performance and measure progress in therapy. Kielhofner emphasized the fact that MOHO-based tools may be used in conjunction with other non-MOHO tools, based on client need and the desired outcomes of the tool.

Intervention techniques within MOHO are aimed at facilitating occupational participation. Kielhofner (2008) identified *occupational participation* as engagement in work, play, or activities of daily living that are part of one's "sociocultural context and are desired and/or necessary to one's well-being" (p. 101). In the current OT Practice Framework (AOTA, 2020), the concept of occupation is expanded to include areas such as religious and spiritual activities, health management, and sleep/rest. Goal development and intervention within MOHO consider the aspects of the person (volition, habituation, and performance capacity), along with the social and physical environment. Therapy focuses on choice of modalities and approach to positively influence an individual's feeling, doing, and thinking to enhance occupational participation and occupational performance. Cole and Tufano (2020) identified the following strategies that may be used in intervention within MOHO:

1. *Validating*: Providing validation, respect and acknowledgement for the client experience
2. *Identifying*: Providing the client information on personal and environmental options and resources

3. *Giving feedback*: Communicating about the client's situation
4. *Advising*: Providing goals and strategies for realistic outcomes (it is important to note this is done in collaboration with the client in order to remain client centered)
5. *Negotiating*: Open communication in a give and take manner regarding future plans
6. *Structuring*: Setting ground rules and clear expectations for performance
7. *Coaching*: Using of prompts and cues for assistance, support, and instruction
8. *Encouraging*: Providing emotional support and reassurance
9. Providing physical support.

The client and the therapist work together to not only set goals and develop the intervention plan, but also to reassess and consider therapy outcomes and future plans.

Summary

Since the founding of occupational therapy, the importance of enabling meaningful doing, or *occupation*, has been the implied purpose of therapeutic interactions. This chapter reviewed important occupation-based models used to guide the occupational therapy process. Although each model is slightly different in approach, common concepts of the models include the *person, environment, occupation*, and influences on *occupational performance*. Occupational therapy uses occupation as a means, and an end, to help individuals throughout their lifespans achieve their full potentials and maintain the highest possible levels of health and well-being.

BOX 7.1 THE POINT IS:

- Common to occupation-based models are the individual *person*, the context including *environmental factors*, the *occupation*, and the resulting *occupational performance*.
- The level of occupational performance depends on the goodness of fit between the person, contextual factors, and occupation.
- Occupation-based models provide a framework for understanding and using occupation in the occupational therapy process.
- Occupation may be used as a means and an end in occupational therapy.

References

American Occupational Therapy Association (AOTA). (2020). Occupational therapy practice framework: Domain and process (4th ed.). *American Journal of Occupational Therapy, 74*(Suppl. 2), 7412410010. https://doi.org/10.5014/ajot.2020.74S2001

Baptiste, S. (2018). Person–environment–occupation model. In J. Hinojosa, P. Kramer, & C. Royeen (Eds.), *Perspectives on human occupation: Theories underlying practice* (2nd ed., pp. 1370159). F. A. Davis.

Baron, K., Kielhofner, G., Iyengar, A., Goldhammer, V., & Wolenski, J. (2006). *Occupational Self-Assessment* (OSA–v. 2.2). University of Illinois Chicago.

Bass, J. D., Baum, C. M., & Christiansen, C. H. (2015). Interventions and outcomes. The person–environment–occupation–performance (PEOP) occupational therapy process. In C. H. Christiansen, C. M. Baum, & J. D. Bass (Eds.), *Occupational therapy: Performance, participation and well-being* (4th ed., pp. 57–80). Slack.

Baum, C. M., Christiansen, C. H., & Bass, J. D. (2015). The person–environment–occupation–performance (PEOP) model. In C. H. Christiansen, C. M. Baum, & J. D. Bass (Eds.), *Occupational therapy: Performance, participation and well-being* (4th ed., pp. 49–55). Slack.

Baum, C. M., & Edwards, D. (2008). *Activity card sort* (2nd ed.). Washington University.

Brown, C. (2019). Ecological models in occupational therapy. In B. A. Schell & G. Gillen (Eds.), *Willard & Spackman's occupational therapy* (13th ed., pp. 622–632). Wolters Kluwer.

Christiansen, C. H., & Baum, C. M (Eds.). (1991). *Occupational therapy: Overcoming human performance deficits*. Slack.

Christiansen, C. H., Baum, C. M, & Bass, J. D. (Eds.). (2015). *Occupational therapy: Performance, participation and well-being*. Slack.

Cole, M. B., & Tufano, R. (2020). *Applied theories in occupational therapy: A practical approach*. Slack.

Cutchin, M. P. (2004). Using Deweyan philosophy to rename and reframe adaptation-to-environment. *American Journal of Occupational Therapy, 58,* 303–312.

de las Heras, C. G., Geist, R., Kielhofner, G., & Yaning, L. (2007). *Volitional questionnaire* (v. 4.1). University of Illinois Chicago.

George, L. A., Schkade, J. K., & Ishee, J. H. (2004). Content validity of the relative mastery measurement scale: A measure of occupational adaptation. *OTJR: Occupation, Participation & Health, 24,* 92–102. https://doi.org/10.5014/ajot.46.10 .91710.1177/153944920402400303

Grajo, L. C. (2019). The theory of occupational adaptation. In B. A. Schell & G. Gillen (Eds.), *Willard & Spackman's occupational therapy* (13th ed., pp. 633–642). Wolters Kluwer.

Grajo, L. C., Boisselle, A., & DaLomba, E. (2018). Occupational adaptation as a construct: A scoping review of literature. *The Open Journal of Occupational Therapy, 6*(2). https://doi.org/10.15453/2168-6408.1400

Gray, J. (1998). Putting occupation into practice: Occupation as ends, occupation as means. *American Journal of Occupational Therapy, 52,* 354–364. https://doi.org/10 .5014/ajot.52.5.354

Kielhofner, G. (1985). *A model of human occupation: Theory and application*. Williams & Wilkins.

Kielhofner, G. (2008). *Model of Human Occupation: Theory and application* (4th ed.). Wolters Kluwer.

Kielhofner, G., & Burke, J. (1980). A model of human occupation, part one. Conceptual framework and content. *American Journal of Occupational Therapy, 34,* 777–788. https://doi.org/10.5014/ajot.34.9.572

Kielhofner, G., & Forsyth, K. (2008). Therapeutic reasoning: Planning, implementing and evaluating the outcomes of therapy. In G. Kielhofner (Ed.), *Model of human occupation: Theory and application* (4th ed., pp. 155–170).

Kielhofner, G., Malinson, T., Crawford, C., Nowak, M., Rigby, M., Henry, A., & Walens, D. (2004). *Occupational performance history interview (OPHI-II)*. University of Illinois Chicago.

Law, M., Baptiste, S., Carswell, A. McColl, M. A., & Pollock, N. (2014). *Canadian occupational performance measure* (5th ed.). Canadian Occupational Therapy Association.

Law, M., Baptiste, S., McColl, M., Opzoomer, A., Polatajko, H., & Pollock, N. (1990). The Canadian occupational performance measure: An outcome measure for occupational therapy. *Canadian Journal of Occupational Therapy, 57*, 82–87. https://doi.org/10.1177/000841749005700207

Law, M., Cooper, B., Strong, S., Stewart, D., Rigby, P., & Letts, L. (1996). The person–environment–occupation model: A transactive approach to occupational performance. *Canadian Journal of Occupational Therapy, 63*, 9–23. https://doi.org/10.1177/000841749606300103

Law, M., & Laver-Fawcett, A. (2013). Canadian model of occupational performance: 30 years of impact! *British Journal of Occupational Therapy, 76*, 519. https://doi.org/10.4276/030802213X13861576675123

McColl, M. A. (2015) Occupation-focused models. In M. A. McColl, M. C. Law, & D. Stewart (Eds.), *Theoretical basis of occupational therapy* (3rd ed., pp. 53–68). Slack.

McColl, M. A., Law, M. C., & Stewart, D. (Eds.) (2015). *Theoretical basis of occupational therapy* (3rd ed.). Slack.

Parkinson, S., Forsyth, K., & Kielhofner, G. (2006). *The model of human occupation screening tool* (MOHOST v. 2). University of Illinois Chicago.

Reed, K. D., Hocking, C. S., & Smythe, L. A. (2011). Exploring the meaning of occupation: The case for phenomenology. *Canadian Journal of Occupational Therapy, 78*, 303–310. https://doi.org/10.2182/cjot.2011.78.5.5

Reid, H. A., Hocking, C., & Smythe, L. (2019). The making of occupation-based models and diagrams: History and semiotic analysis. *Canadian Journal of Occupational Therapy, 86*(4), 313–325. https://doi.org/10.1177/0008417419833413

Reilly, M. (1962). Occupational therapy can be one of the great ideas of 20th century medicine. *American Journal of Occupational Therapy, 16*, 1–9

Johnson, K. R, & Dickie, V. (2019). What is occupation? In B. A. Schell & G. Gillen (Eds.), *Willard & Spackman's occupational therapy* (13th ed., pp. 2–10). Wolters Kluwer.

Rogers, J. C. (1983). Eleanor Clarke Slagle Lectureship—1983; Clinical reasoning: The ethics, science, and art. *The American Journal of Occupational Therapy, 37*(9), 601–616.

Schell, B. B., Gillen, G., & Scaffa, M. (2014). *Willard & Spackman's occupational therapy* (12th ed.). Wolters Kluwer.

Schkade, J. K., & Schultz, S. (1992a). Occupational adaptation: Toward a holistic approach to contemporary practice (part 1). *American Journal of Occupational Therapy, 45*, 829–837. https://doi.org/10.5014/ajot.46.9.829

Schkade, J. K., & Schultz, S. (1992b). Occupational adaptation: Toward a holistic approach to contemporary practice (part 2). *American Journal of Occupational Therapy*, *45*, 917–926. https://doi.org/10.5014/ajot.46.10.917

Schkade, J. K., & Schultz, S. (2003). Occupational adaptation. In P. Kramer, J. Hinojosa, & C. B. Royeen (Eds.), *Perspectives in human occupation: Participation in life* (pp. 181–221). Lippincott Williams & Wilkins.

Schultz, S. (2014). Theory of occupational adaptation. In B. Schell, G. Gillen, & M. Scaffa (Eds.), *Willard & Spackman's occupational therapy* (12th ed., pp. 527–540). Lippincott Williams & Wilkins.

Strong, S. & Reberio-Gruhl, K. (2019). Person–environment–occupation model. In C. Brown, V. C. Stoffel, & J. P. Munoz (Eds.), *Occupational therapy in mental health: A vision for participation* (2nd ed., pp. 29–46). F.A. Davis.

Taylor, R. R. (2017). *Kielhofner's model of human occupation* (5th ed.). Wolters Kluwer.

Townsend, E., & Polatajko, H. (2007). *Enabling occupation II: Advancing an occupational therapy vision for health, well-being and justice through occupation.* CAOT Publications.

Townsend, E., & Polatajko, H. (2013). *Enabling occupation II: A Canadian perspective.* CAOT Publications.

Woodside, H. (1976) Dimensions of the occupational behavior model. *Canadian Journal of Occupational Therapy*, *43*(1), 11–14. https://doi.org/10.1177/000841747604300103

Chapter 8

Introduction to Occupation-based Evaluation

Introduction

An **occupation-based evaluation** requires the therapist to view the client through an occupational lens. Understanding the client perspective, daily occupational patterns, and personal meaning, along with strengths and needs in relation to occupational performance is integral to evaluation. Through engagement in the therapeutic relationship with the client, occupational therapists seek to enable occupational participation in meaningful life tasks within society. The occupational therapy process emphasizes the importance of (a) developing an occupational profile, (b) analysis of values, meaning, participation, and occupational performance (evaluation), (c) the formation of occupation-based goals, (d) intervention, and (e) re-evaluation.

Occupational therapists use a wide range of evaluation methods and assessment tools to guide intervention. This chapter outlines key concepts and considerations for occupation-based evaluation. The principles outlined and assessments included in the chapter will provide an overview of key considerations and general principles for assessment selection and administration.

Principles of Occupation-based Evaluation

The literature varies with respect to definitions and terminology related to occupation-based therapy. This text will refer to Ann Fisher's work, which distinguished among occupation-focused, occupation-centered, and occupation-based occupational therapy. Fisher (2014) asserted each of these has a distinct definition contributing to the understanding of occupation. She identified *occupation-centered* as guiding reasoning and actions in occupational therapy and *occupation-based* and *occupation-focused* as influencing what and how people do what they do in research, education, and practice. Each of these terms has different but related definitions (Fisher, 2014, p. 101):

> *Occupation-centered:* To adopt a profession-specific perspective—a world view of occupation and what it means to be an occupational being—where

DOI: 10.4324/9781003242185-8

occupation is placed in the center and ensures that what practitioners do is linked to the core paradigm of occupational therapy.

Occupation-based: To use occupation as the foundation—to engage a person in occupation (i.e. the performance of chosen daily life tasks that offer desirable levels of pleasure, productivity, and restoration, and unfold as they ordinarily do in the person's life) as the method used for evaluation and/or intervention.

Occupation-focused: To focus attention on occupation—to have occupation as the proximal (i.e. immediate) focus of the evaluation or the proximal intent of the intervention.

Although related, each of these terms provides unique application to occupational therapy. The profession at its core is occupation-centered and influenced by the science of occupation, which distinguishes occupational therapy from other rehabilitation, health, and social science professions. Practitioners use occupation-based methods when they include occupational engagement in their evaluation and intervention. For example, consider that a home-health therapist conducts a kitchen evaluation in a client's apartment. In this instance, the observation and analysis of the occupation and occupational engagement would be considered occupation-based, given that the outcome is based on performance analysis of a client performing a daily occupation.

An occupation-focused approach to assessment has occupation at the core but may or may not involve an actual performance of the task (Asaba et al., 2017). For example, a therapist performing an interview on the client's perspective of occupational performance and areas of need, would be considered occupation-focused, in that occupation is addressed; however, an actual observation of the client engaged in the task (e.g., laundry) is not performed. When possible, it is important to combine evaluation methods such as client and caregiver interview and chart review along with assessment tools that use observation and actual task performance.

As with key concepts of occupation-based models discussed in the previous chapter, evaluation focuses on the *person, environment/context, occupation,* and subsequent *occupational performance.* The Occupational Therapy Practice Framework 4th edition (American Occupational Therapy Association, 2020) identifies the central focus of the occupational therapy process as "achieving health, well-being, and participation in life through engagement in occupation" (p. 5). Evaluation methods include both client and caregiver perspectives on priorities and perceived performance of occupations along with actual observation of a client's occupational performance in order to develop goals and strategies for intervention.

Contextual considerations in the evaluation process include not only the environment in which the client lives, but also the situational context in which the assessment is performed. James and Pitonyak (2019) identified contextual aspects influencing evaluation to include the physical context (whether the assessment is performed in natural or clinical environment) and the social context (e.g., the fact that a client is being observed and evaluated). The authors identified additional evaluation considerations including the safety of the assessment process, the client's background and experience, available resources, time constraints, the practitioner's training and experience, and requirements from organizational policies and/or payment providers. Although performing an assessment in the natural environment (e.g., the client's home or living setting) may be advantageous for a variety of reasons, it is not always practical or feasible to do this. Therefore, therapists must use clinical reasoning to consider client needs and values, environmental factors, and appropriate tools and methods for the evaluation process.

As the therapist and client collaborate in the evaluation process, key questions and considerations must be addressed, as shown in Box 8.1.

BOX 8.1 KEY QUESTIONS AND CONSIDERATIONS IN OCCUPATION-BASED EVALUATION

1. What is the purpose of the evaluation?
2. How will the evaluation support occupational performance?
3. What occupation-based and occupation-focused evaluation methods and assessment tools are available?
4. What are the psychometric properties (reliability and validity) of the tools selected and are they appropriate to the client's age, needs, purpose of the assessment, ability to participate in the assessment, and the practitioner's training?
5. What are the client's values, interests, strengths, needs, and priorities?
6. What is the training of the practitioner?
7. How will the dynamic of the provider–client relationship affect the evaluation results?
8. What are the resources and time considerations (e.g., how long will the client receive services)?
9. Who is paying for services and are there parameters and policies governing the evaluation process (e.g., insurer, facility, or assessment training requirements)?
10. What occupations give meaning to the client and how will the evaluation support occupation-based goal planning and intervention?
11. Will results of the evaluation process translate to the client's natural environment (e.g., support occupational performance in the home)?
12. Is there a plan for re-evaluation and follow-up?

The practitioner uses clinical reasoning throughout the occupational therapy process to respond to the client's needs and any changes that may occur. For instance, if an individual with a right CVA who is working with a therapist on regaining dressing skills has a medical setback, the therapist, client, and team will determine changes necessary to the evaluation and intervention plan in order to best meet the client's needs.

The Evaluation Process and Assessment Tools

There are several reasons an evaluation is performed. In addition to the evaluation process that occurs upon admission, assessment tools may be used to consider current occupational performance, measure response to intervention (evaluation/re-evaluation), for consultative purposes, and to facilitate decision making regarding discharge planning. The evaluation process extends beyond the scores of an individual assessment tool to include the history, reason for referral, client and contextual factors, and client and family perceptions, values, and priorities. The following is a brief description of the evaluation process along with a discussion of sample occupation-focused and occupation-based assessment tools.

Occupational Profile

The evaluation process begins with the development of an **occupational profile**. According to the Practice Framework (AOTA, 2020), "the occupational profile is a summary of a client's (person's, group's, or population's) occupational history and experiences, patterns of daily living, interests, values, needs, and relevant contexts" (p. 21). The occupational profile views the client as an occupational being and is designed to identify the occupational areas the client wishes to work on and areas that may impede performance (Whitney, 2019). As part of the process, the practitioner interviews the client and uses reflective listening skills and clinical reasoning to fully understand the person's story and how that may influence the intervention process. The client's narrative provides an understanding of how the past and present influence future goals and may provide insights into how the client, environment, and occupation impede or facilitate occupational performance (Mattingly, 1994; Unsworth, 2004). Questions asked include why the client is seeking or referred for services; how the client perceives strengths and limitations to occupational performance; what are the individual's values and priorities; what is the client's occupational history; and how do existing performance patterns influence occupational engagement. Additional questions may be related to how specific client or contextual factors may influence performance. Therapists may choose to use a formalized occupational profile template (e.g., those provided by a professional association), or summarize the information narratively in preparation for the analysis of occupational performance.

Assessment Tools

Once the occupational profile is established, practitioners use clinical reasoning along with evidence to select assessment tools suited to the client. Although concepts of occupation-based assessment differ in the literature, Hocking (2001) emphasized the importance of considering humans as occupational beings and occupation as involving meaning, function, form, and performance components. Thus, consideration of the client's occupational goals along with the purpose of the occupation and how it contributes to personal identity is relevant to the selection and administration of the assessment tool. Assessments may be occupation-based and include actual performance of the occupation or may be occupation-focused and involve interviews and other methods designed to understand the client's concept and value of the occupation.

Research indicates that performance-based assessments have greater ecological validity and thus provide a clearer indication of the client's abilities in their customary performance settings (Edwards et al., 2019). For example, an individual with a recent traumatic brain injury showing cognitive difficulties may report that they are able to perform certain IADLs. Yet, when they are asked to demonstrate these tasks in a home-based assessment, they may show difficulties with sequencing, judgment, and following directions. Thus, a combination of assessment approaches is helpful in the evaluation process. Once the key questions posed earlier are considered (see Box 8.1), the specific assessments and appropriate environment(s) for completing the evaluation can be more effectively chosen.

Evaluation and intervention approaches may be top down or bottom up. Trombly (1993) identified the top-down approach to include the occupation, meaning, and roles of the client as the initial primary focus, with the foundational skills, performance patterns, and activity demands considered later. She identified the bottom-up approach as focusing "on the deficits of components of function, such as strength, range of motion, balance, and so on, which are believed to be prerequisites to successful occupational performance or functioning" (Trombly, 1993, p. 253). Although there is often overlap in the occupational therapy process and practitioners use both approaches, occupation-based and **occupation-focused assessment** tools and models generally use a top-down approach. Therefore, in a rehabilitation department, an occupation-based top-down approach to evaluation would not emphasize individual muscle testing of the upper extremity, but rather may include an observation of a client performing a kitchen task. Although there is practical benefit to both top-down and bottom-up approaches, the consideration of the occupation, environment, person, and subsequent occupational performance is the main focus of the occupation-based top-down approach. Consideration should be given to the practical application of the findings to the client's everyday environment. Although the top-down approach emphasizes occupation at its core, it is important to also consider

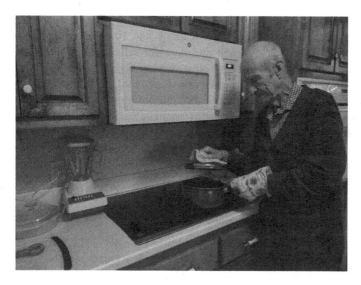

Figure 8.1 Occupation-based evaluation includes actual observation of task performance, preferably in the setting where tasks are typically performed. Research supports the value of using performance-based assessments (photo courtesy of Kristine Haertl)

underlying performance skills and needs that affect (inhibit or restrict) occupational performance. The following presents a sample of occupation-based and occupation-focused assessment tools.

Canadian Occupational Performance Measure (COPM)

The Canadian Occupational Performance Measure (Law et al., 1994, 2014) is a client-centered tool used to identify client and caregiver needs and priorities. This tool measures the client's perception of occupational performance and personal priorities in the areas of self-care, productivity, and leisure. The COPM includes both roles and role expectations within the client's living environment through an individualized interview approach that takes about 15-30 minutes to perform (Law et al., 2005). The administration of this assessment involves a five-step process:

- Problem identification/definition
- Initial assessment
- Occupational therapy intervention
- Reassessment
- Calculation of change.

Once areas of concern are identified, the client is asked to rate the importance of each activity on a scale of 1 to 10. The client or caregiver then rates the client's ability in each of these areas on a scale of 1 to 10. The scale results in two scores, one for performance and the other for satisfaction. Therapists then work collaboratively with the client on **goal planning**, intervention, and plans for reassessment. Since this is an interview-based tool, the authors advise that additional assessment of performance through observation and standardized assessment helps provide a more holistic (complete) analysis of the client's strengths, needs, values, and performance. The updated COPM is available in 35 languages, and may be used with both clients and families to identify priorities, goals, and client–caregiver perceptions of change over time (Canadian Occupational Performance Measure, 2022).

Assessment of Motor and Process Skills (AMPS)

The Assessment of Motor and Process Skills (AMPS) (Fisher, 1989; Fisher & Jones, 2014) is a standardized observational tool that measures a person's performance capacity in several ADL and IADL tasks. The assessment begins with a client interview and proceeds to evaluate a client's quality of performance through rating the effort, efficiency, safety, and independence on a task. Two scales are used to separately measure motor and process skills. During the task performance of each of the 16 motor and 20 process skills, the client is rated on a four-point scale: 1= *deficit*, 2= *ineffective*, 3= *questionable*, and 4= *competent*. Scores are entered into a computer and a comprehensive report is generated to help identify levels of ability and priorities for intervention. Given the complexity of the assessment, therapists are required to complete a certification process in order to administer the AMPS. The assessment tool is widely used internationally and may be useful for initial evaluation, as well as measurement of change following intervention.

Model of Human Occupation Tools

The Model of Human Occupation (MOHO) has several interview and observational tools available across the lifespan, many of which are available at the MOHO Clearinghouse at www.moho.uic.edu/. The following are examples and brief descriptions of tools available:

Model of Human Occupation Screening Tool (MOHOST): The MOHOST (Parkinson et al., 2006) has 24 items that measure key concepts of MOHO including volition, habituation, skills, and environment. Therapists may use a variety of data sources such as an interview, chart review, caregiver report, and observation in order to rate the client on motivation for occupation, patterns of occupation, communication and interaction skills, process skills, motor skills, and the environment. Each item is rated based on a FAIR scale (F—facilitates occupation, A—allows occupational participation, I—inhibits occupation, and R—restricts occupation). The summary includes an analysis of strengths and limitations and may be used in goal planning and measurement of change over time. As a tool widely used in mental health and other practice settings, research has demonstrated its value as well as the importance of adequate training prior to administration (Bugajska & Brooks, 2021). Use of the measure at regular intervals may also serve for future goal setting and intervention planning and to justify services.

Occupational Self-Assessment (OSA) and Child Occupational Self-Assessment: The OSA (Baron et al., 2006) and COSA (Kramer et al., 2014) assessments are designed to elicit the client's perspective on occupational competence in a variety of occupational activities. Within the OSA, clients rate themselves on a four-point scale as to how well they perform the activity and the importance of each. The client and therapist then work together to form goals for therapy. The COSA is a similar instrument adapted for the pediatric population and thus rather than a rating scale, young clients give feedback via use of smiley and frowning faces related to performance. Two frowning faces indicate a "big problem," one indicates a "little problem," a smiling face indicates the client does the activity "ok," and two smiling faces indicates "I am really good at doing this." Similarly, stars are used to indicate the importance of the activity from one star "not really important to me," to four stars, "most important of all to me." Within these assessments, there is a short form available of the OSA if there are time constraints or if it is to be used with more lengthy observational tools. In both assessments, the client's perspective is a key element of planning intervention.

Assessment of Communication and Interaction Skills (ACIS): The ACIS (Forsyth et al., 1998) is a formal observational tool that observes clients in a structured group situation performing a specific task within a context that is relevant to the client. Such observations may occur in a task group within therapy, or in a naturalistic environment such as a client interacting with family members in the home. The unique feature of this tool is that it assesses communication and interaction with consideration of the occupational form and the context. The therapist performs the observation in an environmental situation closely similar to that in which the task is usually performed. The ACIS has 20 skill items that are divided into three separate communication and interaction domains, including physicality, information exchange, and relations. Sample items in *physicality* include contacts, gazes, orients, and postures, items within the *information exchange* domain include areas such as articulates, asks, asserts, expresses, and engages, and examples of the *relations* section include collaborates, conforms, focuses, relates, and respects. Clients are rated on a 4-point scale (4=competent; 3=questionable, 2=ineffective, and 1=deficit). Results are used in collaboration with the client to determine strengths and needs in communication and interaction. Since ratings are on communication and interaction, clinical reasoning skills are required to rate the client in comparison to societal norms and expectations within the context of the occupation performed.

Volitional Questionnaire (VQ) and Pediatric Volitional Questionnaire (PVQ): The VQ (de las Heras et al., 2007) and PVQ (Basu et al., 2008) assessments are observational measures. The assessment may occur in a natural environment or within the context of a therapy session and provides structured analysis of how the client acts within the environment and how motivation is affected. Examples of volitional items rated include "shows curiosity," "tries new things," and "seeks challenges." Items are rated as P—passive, H—hesitant, I—involved, or S—spontaneous. Results provide information on the client's motivational strengths, needs, and environmental supports in occupational performance. Information from the VQ and PVQ can be used to identify environmental influences on motivation, volition (motivation) within occupational tasks, and to identify intrinsic motivational changes over time.

Work Environment Impact Scale (WEIS) (Moore-Corner et al., 1998) and *Worker Role Interview* (Braveman et al., 2005): There are a number of interview and observational tools to assess the client's function at the work place as well as the client–environment fit. The WEIS is a 17-item semi-structured interview and rating scale designed to assess how clients with psychosocial, cognitive, and physical disabilities experience their work environments. The interview examines physical and social aspects of the work environment along with specific task demands and objects used. Clients need to have the capacity for self-awareness and the ability to participate in an interview using a rating scale. The WEIS has been used to measure employee sustainability (Qing et al., 2021) and has demonstrated good reliability and validity. This tool may be used with the Worker Role Interview and/or additional observation-based work assessments. The Worker Role Interview is a semi-structured set of questions that includes a 16-item scale that measures personal causation, values, interests, roles, habits, and environment. It is designed for those out of work due to injury or disability and measures on a scale from SS=Strongly supports client returning to job, to SI=Strongly interferes with returning to job. Insights from the interview can inform future work plans as well as interventions designed to facilitate return to work.

Additional tools: There are several other occupation-focused and occupation-based tools in areas of occupation including basic activities of daily living (BADL), instrumental activities of daily living (IADL), education/work, play/leisure, social participation, and rest/sleep. For instance, therapists may choose the *Kohlman Evaluation of Living Skills* (KELS) (Kohlman-Thomson & Robnett, 2016), or the *Performance Assessment of Self-Care Skills* (PASS) (Holm, 2020) as performance-based tools to assess ADL and IADL; a child play scale such as the *Revised Knox Preschool Play Scale* (Knox, 1997) to assess play in the pediatric population; or the *School Function Assessment* (Coster et

Table 8.1 A selected list of occupation-based and occupation-focused assessment tools

Assessment name	Population	Description	Time required
Assessment of Communication and Interaction Skills	Adults	Observational assessment on an activity requiring communication and social interaction	20–60 minutes
Assessment of Motor and Process Skills (AMPS)	3 years–adult	Observational task assessment that requires therapist training	30–60 minutes
Canadian Occupational Performance Measure	Children with a mental age of 8–adult	Interview tool that measures perceived satisfaction and performance in self-care, productivity and leisure	20–60 minutes
Kohlman Evaluation of Living Skills	Adults	Interview and observational tool in ADL, IADL, and communication	30–60 minutes
Knox Preschool Play Scale	Infants and children 0–6 years	Observational rating scale based on standardized behaviors	Often performed in two 30-minute play sessions indoors or outdoors.
Model of Human Occupation Screening Tool (MOHOST)	Adults	Screening tool using multiple means of data collection: Interview, chart review, observation to assess performance	10–40 minutes
Occupational Self-Assessment (OSA) and Child Occupational Self-Assessment (COSA)	Adults (OSA) Children (COSA)	Self-rating assessments related to everyday occupational activities. Clients must have capacity for self-assessment	OSA: 15–35 minutes COSA: 35–45 minutes
Performance Assessment of Self Care Skills (PASS)	Age 13 years and higher	Observational performance based tool of ADL & IADL	1.5–3 hours
School Functional Assessment	Children K-6 (5–12 years)	Questionnaire for teachers on client's school performance	1.5–2 hours

(Continued)

Table 8.1 (Continued)

Assessment name	Population	Description	Time required
Volitional Questionnaire (VQ) and Pediatric Volitional Questionnaire (PVQ) .	Adults Children	Observation of task performance	30 minutes–1 hour
Worker Environment Impact Scale (WEIS)	Adults	Semi-structured interview	30 minutes–1 hour
Worker Role Interview	Adults	Semi-structured interview	30 minutes–1 hour

al., 1998) to assess performance in a school setting. The focus of these tools is to identify strengths, needs, and priorities in occupational performance. Table 8.1 provides a selected list of occupation-focused and occupation-based tools used in practice. There are several additional tools available for individuals across the lifespan.

In summary, consideration of occupation as integral to the selection of assessment tools includes asking the key questions presented earlier (in Box 8.1), along with consideration of whether the assessment will support evaluation and intervention to promote occupational performance in areas of meaning within the client's life. When possible, assessment in natural contexts is best and standardized and non-standardized occupation-focused and occupation-based tools are selected with consideration of client motivation, context/environment, and occupational performance.

Goal Planning

Once the information from the evaluation process is gathered and synthesized, therapists use critical reasoning to create a holistic understanding of the client. It is vitally important that therapeutic reasoning extends beyond the numerical scores of assessment tools, as often there are extenuating circumstances influencing score outcomes that must be considered. For instance, if a client with substance abuse and addiction attains a high score on ADL and IADL assessments, this does not automatically mean the client should be considered for independent living. Additional factors such as the status of the substance condition along with support factors and client needs, strengths, and priorities should also be considered. Information from the evaluation includes the client and contextual factors in forming goals and planning intervention.

BOX 8.2 OCCUPATION IN ACTION: A GROUP HOME SUPPORTED WORK SETTING

In addition to a role as a professor, the author of this case description (KH) maintains a private practice working with clients who have developmental and mental health conditions. It is common to receive referrals for evaluations that focus only on performance skills without consideration of the impact on the client's occupational engagement. Occasionally, a referral may arrive to assess a client's sensory processing or cognition. It is appropriate to educate referral sources that this practice uses a holistic approach toward evaluation that includes consideration of the client (*person*), context (*environment*), daily activity requirements and demands (*occupations*), and performance. Although consideration of performance skills is important in an occupation-based evaluation, a top-down approach provides insight related to current strengths and needs in daily performance.

CASE EXAMPLE

Shane is a 28-year-old male with anxiety, depression, and moderate intellectual disability. He recently had increased difficulty focusing on his work program and engaged in self-injurious and assaultive behaviors. He was at risk for losing his valued position working in a supported employment warehouse. Shane's referral requested a sensory processing assessment. Upon talking with staff at the group home and reviewing records, it was apparent that a more thorough top-down assessment of the work environment, Shane's strengths and needs, and his personal interests be included in the evaluation. The occupation-based assessment included not only performance skill-based tools, but also a client interview, use of the *Work Environment Impact Scale*, and occupational observation in the work role. While the use of only a sensory processing tool may have provided valuable information, the occupation-based evaluation components allowed for additional insights. These revealed that Shane worked in a busy, noisy room that increased his anxiety and difficulties with sensory processing. Although the client was highly skilled in his sorting tasks, he struggled to concentrate in his work environment. Within the interview he demonstrated insight into his anxiety and agreed that a quieter environment would help. Following the evaluation, potential work modifications were discussed with Shane and his vocational support staff. Collaboration with the worksite allowed for environmental changes to support improved performance, decreased anxiety, and fewer difficult behaviors. The client was placed in a room with fewer individuals, was given breaks when needed, and used headphones with his favorite music to decrease external noise. Within a month his behaviors and work performance improved and he was able to keep the position he values.

Application Questions:

1. What concepts of occupation-based evaluation are demonstrated in this example?
2. What were the advantages of a top-down approach to evaluation in this situation?

Following the evaluation process and development of a holistic representation of the individual being assessed, therapists collaborate to the extent possible with the client to form goals. Such collaboration may include the client/patient, family members, care givers, and others closely involved in the individual's life. Goal setting should also consider the initial reason for referral as well as prognosis and discharge expectations. Goals should be relevant, valued by the client, focused on function, and measurable (Brown et al., 2019). In an occupation-based approach, goals must also be occupational in nature. For instance, while improvement in balance or strength may be an important subcomponent of a larger goal (e.g., return to work as a gardener), the actual goal should focus on the occupational task. Kielhofner and Forsyth (2008) emphasized the following in goal planning and implementation:

- Working collaboratively to create goals with the client
- Deciding what types of occupational engagement will enable change
- Determining strategies needed to support client change
- Enhancing understanding of performance capacities (both strengths and needs)
- Developing emotional acceptance of limitations and pride in occupational abilities
- Building confidence to approach occupational tasks
- Increasing knowledge and acceptance of using adaptive aids and environmental modifications when needed
- Increasing willingness to ask for help if needed
- Increasing readiness for goal attainment and occupational challenges.

Following goal development, the intervention plan is formed, goals are monitored and re-evaluated, and outcomes are measured. Although the process appears linear, given the dynamic nature of humans, factors influence progress and thus therapists must use clinical reasoning to adapt to the client, environmental, and occupational changes that may occur in the occupational therapy process.

BOX 8.3 OCCUPATION IN AN ACUTE CARE SETTING: CREATING A SENSE OF DOING

In acute care, it is common for occupational therapists to receive orders for discharge planning while a patient has been hospitalized for a chronic condition or acute medical event. As an occupational therapist, an important role is to assist clients and the health care team in creating a sense of doing within an environment that is highly medical in nature. Additional goals include providing an occupation-based picture of the client's current abilities as well as an understanding of the occupational and environmental demands after the hospitalization. Physicians and other health care team members are continually educated about the occupational lens through which an evaluation of the client (person), context (environment), and daily occupational needs of the client must be considered if therapeutic goals are to be achieved.

CASE EXAMPLE

A 78-year-old female was admitted for failure to thrive and respiratory distress with co-morbidities of end-stage heart failure, generalized anxiety, and depression. Prior to being hospitalized, the client lived alone with a weekly check from her daughter. The client is a retired desk clerk and finds meaning in participating in weekly crafting at her church. The referral for OT was requested to evaluate the client based on a perceived decline in self-care performance and increase in depressive symptoms. The client's electronic medical record was reviewed to determine prior levels of function in the home environment, and current function and performance in the hospital (e.g., mobility with nursing). The client's relevant medical status (e.g., surgical procedures, lab tests, vital signs) were also noted. Upon arrival to the room, nursing staff informed the practitioner that the patient was withdrawn and not consistently completing her daily self-care tasks.

The occupation-based approach within the room included a client interview at bedside, assessment of performance skills, and a standardized cognitive and social measure. During the interview the client provided insight into her overall weakness and depressed mood since being in the hospital. A standardized self-care screening tool (e.g., Activity Measure for Post-Acute Care—6 Clicks —Inpatient Daily Activity Short Form) was then used. The client was provided a prompt-assisted opportunity to complete her grooming routine with similar tools and processes used at home. This started with brushing her teeth and washing her face at the sink and concluded with sitting in the bedside recliner for her to groom her hair. During the grooming activity, the client indicated that crafting was a passion and routine activity at home. A leisure-based questionnaire (e.g., Interest Checklist) was used to further understand her interests at home and to identify potential approaches to improving her mood and activity participation while hospitalized. To support this, supplies and instructions on making a small tie blanket were provided. This activity could be completed between therapy sessions to address her depressed mood and engage the client with an occupation of interest—crafting. She found this activity to be new, yet fulfilling. She planned to share the completed tie pillow at the next church craft gathering upon her return home. Occupational therapy staff returned daily until the patient was discharged after a five-day hospital stay. During each session, occupational therapy staff facilitated self-care activities to build activity tolerance with daily self-care and home management, educated her on adaptive strategies to conserve her energy, and promoted activities that supported occupational engagement while hospitalized. After a five-day hospital stay, with daily participation in occupational therapy, the client was able to return home with functional improvements in her daily self-care activities as well as her leisure activity of crafting.

Questions

1. What concepts of occupation-based evaluation are demonstrated in this case example?
2. What are the advantages of a top-down approach to evaluate occupation within a highly medical practice setting?

(Hannah Oldenburg, ED.D., OTR/L, BCPR)

BOX 8.4 OCCUPATION IN ACTION: A CHILD IN AN OLD ORDER AMISH FAMILY

As a pediatric therapist, the author has been fortunate to serve families from richly diverse backgrounds and contexts. This exposure enlightens the professional reasoning process, which ultimately leads to the selection of age-appropriate standardized pediatric evaluations and collaborative goal development. It is in this decision-making space, however, that challenges may occur in identifying an evaluation that balances measurement of *normed* developmental milestones with measurement of *culturally determined* and *contextually derived* developmental milestones. This is especially striking in this therapist's *pro bono* work with Old Order Amish clients, since current standardized pediatric assessments often measure a child's participation as it is influenced by technology, modern conveniences and appliances, transportation, secondary education, or shared public spaces. How might occupational therapists compare child development across centuries (1800s lifestyle vs. current day) or across vastly different family roles, physical spaces, or life course expectations?

CASE EXAMPLE

Tobias is a third-grade student in his one-room Amish schoolhouse. The schoolhouse has approximately 30 students in grades 1–8. His birth and medical history are unremarkable; he has no formal learning disability diagnosis. He does wear glasses at school (which he greatly dislikes). His parents report that Tobias is having difficulty staying focused during school and is struggling with the "3Rs" (reading, writing, and arithmetic). Their primary goal is for Tobias to remember what he has read in his English-language storybook. His primary goal is to "get faster at reading" so he's not embarrassed when his classmates finish before him. Upon meeting and interviewing Tobias and his parents, the therapist decided against administering a norm-referenced literacy scale, as comparing his functional reading ability to age-equivalent, English-speaking, non-Amish children was not desired by the family. Instead, in support of Tobias' student role, a criterion-referenced assessment of functional reading was chosen (and adapted for cultural relevancy) that also served to address his overarching goal to fit in with his classmates. The criterion tool allowed Tobias and his parents to establish a meaningful starting point of functional reading capacity, while also providing the opportunity to track his response to occupational therapy treatment over time. In this way, Tobias' ability to participate in the occupation of functional reading while promoting non-discriminatory and culturally relevant evaluation practices was made possible.

Application Questions

1. When using standardized assessments to evaluate clients in marginalized or underrepresented populations, what should occupational therapists be mindful of?
2. What are the advantages of criterion-referenced evaluation in this unique situation?
3. What subgoals might Tobias and his parents co-create to help make reading more enjoyable?

(Ashlea Cardin, OTD, OTR/L)

Summary

In this chapter, occupation-focused and occupation-based approaches to evaluation are discussed. Effective assessment of occupational performance is important for developing goals and intervention plans. The therapeutic relationship and critical thinking are integral to the evaluation process. Initial data collection includes coming to understand the client through interviews, chart reviews, and observation. Therapists then develop an occupational profile, select assessment tools, synthesize evaluation results, and collaboratively work with the client to develop goals and intervention plans. It is important to maintain open communication with the client, outlining the steps and purpose of the entire process. Regardless of the steps in the process, the therapist always maintains a focus on the client's life situation and the relevance of goals and interventions to that situation.

BOX 8.5 THE POINT IS:

- Occupation-focused evaluation has occupation at its core but may not use a performance-based assessment (e.g., use of the COPM).
- Occupation-based evaluation includes actual performance of a task.
- Occupation-based evaluation uses a top-down approach.
- Contextual factors of the client's anticipated living environment are relevant to the selection of assessment tools.
- Collaborative goal planning uses information from the evaluation, and considers the clients' strengths, needs, values, contextual factors, and expectations for discharge.

Acknowledgment

Appreciation is extended to Dr. Hannah Oldenburg and Dr. Ashlea Cardin for their valued contributions to the preparation of this chapter.

References

American Occupational Therapy Association (AOTA). (2020). Occupational therapy practice framework: Domain and process (4th ed.). *American Journal of Occupational Therapy, 74*(Suppl. 2), 7412410010. https://doi.org/10.5014/ajot.2020.74S2001

Asaba, E., Nakamura, M., Asaba, A., & Kottorp, A. (2017). Integrating occupational therapy specific assessments in practice: Exploring practitioner perspectives. *Occupational Therapy International*, Article 7602805, 1–8. https://doi.org/10.1155/2017/7602805

Baron, K., Kielhofner, G., Iyenger, A., Goldhammer, V., & Wolenski, J. (2006). *The Occupational Self Assessment (OSA)* (v. 2.2). MOHO Clearinghouse.

Basu, S., Kafkes, A., Schatz, R., Kiraly, A., & Kielhofner, G. (2008). *Pediatric Volitional Questionnaire (PVQ)* (v. 2.1). MOHO Clearinghouse.

Braveman, B., Robson, M., Velozo, C., Kielhofner, G., Fisher, G., Forsyth, K., & Kerschbaum, J. (2005). *Worker Role Interview (WR)* (v. 10.0). MOHO Clearinghouse.

Brown, E. V., Munoz, J. P., & Pan, A. (2019). Person-centered evaluation. In C. Brown, V. C. Stoffel, & J. P. Munoz (Eds.), *Occupational therapy in mental health: A vision for participation* (2nd ed., pp. 47–68). F.A. Davis.

Bugajska, K., & Brooks, R. (2021). Evaluating the use of the model of human occupation screening tool in mental health services. *British Journal of Occupational Therapy, 84,* 591–600. https://doi.org/10.1177/0308022620956580

Law, M. C., Baptiste, S., Carswell, A., McColl, M. A., Polatajko, H., & Pollock, N. (1998). *Canadian occupational performance measure: COPM.* CAOT Publ. ACE.

Coster, W., Deeney, T, Haltiwanger, J., & Haley, S. (1998). *School functional assessment.* The Psychological Corporation.

de las Heras, C. G., Geist, R., Kielhofner, G. & Yanling, L. (2007). *Volitional Questionnaire (VQ)* (v. 4.1). MOHO Clearinghouse.

Edwards, D. F., Wolf, T. J., Marks, T., Alter, S., Larkin, V., Padesky, B. L., Spiers, M., Alheizen, M. O., & Giles, G. M. (2019). Reliability and validity of a functional cognition screening tool to identify the need for occupational therapy. *American Journal of Occupational Therapy, 73.* https://doi.org/10.5014/ajot.2019.028753

Fisher, A. G. (1989). *Assessment of motor and process skills.* Three Star Press.

Fisher, A. G. (2014). Occupation-centred, occupation-based, occupation-focused: Same, same or different? *Scandinavian Journal of Occupational Therapy, 21,* 96–107. https://doi.org/10.3109/11038128.2014.952912

Fisher, A. G., & Jones, K. B. (2014). *Assessment of motor and process skills: User manual* (8th ed.). Three Star Press.

Forsyth, K., Salamy, M., Simon, S., & Kielhofner, G. (1998). *The Assessment of Communication and Interaction Skills* (v. 4.0). MOHO Clearinghouse.

Hocking, C. (2001). The issue is: Implementing occupation-based assessment. *American Journal of Occupational Therapy, 55*(4). 463–469. https://doi.org/10.5014/ajot.55.4.463

Holm, M. (2020). *The Performance Assessment of Self Care Skills.* In B. Hemphill & C. Urish (Eds.), *Assessments in occupational mental health: An integrative approach* (4th ed., pp. 359–370). Slack.

James, A. B., & Pitonyak, J. S. (2019). Activities of daily living and instrumental activities of daily living. In B. A. Schell & G. Gillen (Eds.), *Willard & Spackman's occupational therapy* (13th ed., pp. 714 –752). Wolters Kluwer.

Kielhofner, G., & Forsyth, K. (2008). Therapeutic reasoning: Planning, implementing and evaluating the outcomes of therapy. In G. Kielhofner (Ed.), *Model of human occupation: Theory and application* (4th ed., pp. 155–170).

Knox, S. (1997). Development and current use of the Knox Preschool Play Scale. In D. Parham, & L. Fazio (Eds.), *Play in occupational therapy for children* (pp. 35–51). Mosby.

Kohlman-Thomson, L., & Robnett, R. (2016). *Kohlman evaluation of living skills* (4th ed). AOTA Press.

Kramer, J., ten Valden, M., Kafkes, A., Basu, S., Federico, J., & Kielhofner, G. (2014). *Child Occupational Self-Assessment (COSA)* (Version 2.2). MOHO Clearinghouse.

Law, M., Baptiste, S., Carswell, A., McColl, M. A., Polatajko, H., & Pollock, N. (1994). *Canadian Occupational Performance Measure* (2nd ed.). Toronto: CAOT Publications.

Law, M., Baptiste, S., Carswel, A., McColl, M. A., Polatajko, H., & Pollock. N. (2005). *Canadian Occupational Performance Measure* (4th ed). CAOT Publications.

Law, M., Canadian Occupational Therapy Association, et al. (2014). *Canadian Occupational Performance Measure* (5th ed.). CAOT Publications.

Mattingly C (1994b) The narrative nature of clinical reasoning. In C. Mattingly & M. H. Fleming (Eds.), *Clinical reasoning: Forms of inquiry in a therapeutic practice* (pp. 239–269). F. A. Davis.

Moore-Corner, R., Kielhofner, G., & Olson, L. (1998). *Work Environment Impact Scale (WEIS)* (v. 2.0). MOHO Clearinghouse.

Parkinson, S., Forsyth, K., & Kielhofner, G. (2006). *The Model of Human Occupation Screening Tool* (v. 2.0). MOHO Clearinghouse.

Qing, D. S., Minh, K. K., Xin, K. C., YanLin, E. C., Chern, A., Budiharjdo, V., & Tan, B. L. (2021). Using the Work Behavior Inventory and Work Environment Impact Scale to measure employment sustainability for people with severe mental illness in a vocational rehabilitation program. *Australian Occupational Therapy Journal, 68,* 246–256. https://doi.org/10.1111/1440-1630.12718

Trombly, C. (1993) Anticipating the future: Assessment of occupational function. *American Journal of Occupational Therapy, 47,* 253–257. https://doi.org/10.5014/ajot.47.3.253

Unsworth, C. A. (2004). Clinical reasoning: How do pragmatic reasoning, worldview and client-centeredness fit? *British Journal of Occupational Therapy, 67*(1), 10–19. https://doi.org/10.1177/030802260406700103

Whitney, R. (2019). *The occupational profile as a guide to clinical reasoning in early intervention: A detective's tale.* AOTA CE article April 2019, CEA0419.

Chapter 9

Introduction to Occupation-based Intervention

Introduction

The core focus of occupational therapy intervention includes the promotion of health, well-being, and participation through occupation. A study of experts published in 2021 and summarized in Chapter 1 unanimously agreed that recognizing the relationship between occupation and health (and well-being) was the most important occupational science concept for occupational therapists to know (Backman et al., 2021). The means through which therapists collaborate with clients to achieve goals to improve health and well-being varies, as do perceptions of what constitutes occupation-based intervention. Chapter 8 introduced the reader to Fisher's (2014) differentiation between occupation-centered, occupation-focused, and occupation-based terminology. This chapter will further explore the terminology, present criteria from the literature used to describe occupation-based intervention (OBI), and will discuss interventions appropriate to individuals, groups, and populations. The chapter will conclude with a brief discussion on **therapeutic use of self** and its relevance to occupation-based practice.

Considerable evidence exists related to the positive health benefits of participation in meaningful occupation (e.g., Gallagher et al., 2015; Ikiugu et al., 2018). Ikiugu et al. (2018) suggested this in part is due to the positive feelings derived from meaningful occupations. The connection between occupation and health is fundamental to occupational therapy, yet conceptualizations of OT interventions grounded in occupation vary in the literature. The AOTA Practice Framework 4th edition (2020) identifies the central focus of its domain and process as "achieving health, well-being, and participation in life through engagement in occupation" (p. 5). Within occupational therapy approaches to intervention, the 2020 edition of the Framework identified preparatory methods of intervention as "interventions to support occupation," which infers that even an intervention procedure that may not be inherently occupational (e.g., splinting), may be used to support enhanced occupational performance. Thus, there is a wide variety of modalities occupational therapists use to facilitate occupational

DOI: 10.4324/9781003242185-9

performance. For the purposes of this chapter, consideration will be given to the following:

- **Occupation-focused** and **occupation-based intervention**
- **Top-down** and **bottom-up approaches**
- **Occupation as a means and an end**
- Factors influencing occupation (e.g., client factors; context; meaning)
- Individual, groups, and systems approaches.

Occupation-based intervention (OBI) includes a broad definition of the term *client* to refer not only to individuals, but to groups, populations, and systems as well. Thus, occupation-focused service delivery from an occupational therapist may include individual intervention approaches such as facilitating return to work as an administrative assistant following a hand injury or working from a systems perspective with a group home on environmental redesign to promote occupational participation for the residents. Thus, in occupation-focused and occupation-based therapy, occupation is central, regardless of the type of client, service delivery, or method used.

Intervention Approaches

Previous chapters discussed the importance of the *person, environment*, and subsequent *occupational performance*, along with various models and approaches to evaluation. Once the occupational profile and evaluation process are completed and goals identified, the therapist works with the client to determine the plan for intervention. Gillen (2019) asserted that intervention should be client-centered, evidenced-based, and grounded in professional reasoning. It is important to note that evidenced-based practice (EBP) not only refers to the research available, but includes (a), the best available evidence, (b), the therapist's knowledge and skills based on previous experience, and (c) the client's wishes, needs, and values. In addition to understanding the client's views within the evaluation process, incorporation of EBP must also include the client's occupational priorities (Occupational Therapy Australia, 2018).

There are varying levels of evidence that are considered along with cultural differences and multiple ways of knowing when providing intervention. Along with evidence from the research literature, confidence, trust, beliefs, personal values, and intuition are all relevant to the therapy process. For instance, while it is straightforward to measure range of motion, or performance on an objective test, client characteristics such as belief, self-esteem, and value may be more readily explored through interviews, observation, qualitative methods, and other approaches. The therapist uses both the art and science of therapy to work with the client and determine the most appropriate method. The therapist comes to know the client through their story or *narrative*. Thus, when using EBP in intervention, the therapist considers the evidence, the client's values, and uses clinical reasoning when selecting specific methods and approaches for intervention. The Occupational Therapy Practice Framework (AOTA, 2020) identifies intervention approaches to include:

- *Create/Promote (health promotion)*—provides contextual and activity/ occupation experiences for enhanced performance
- *Establish/Restore (remediation/restoration)*—addressing underlying client variables affecting performance (often bottom up)
- *Maintain*—preservation of occupational performance
- *Modify*—revision of context or activity to enhance occupational performance
- *Prevent*—directed toward preventing barriers and hindrances to occupational performance.

Table 9.1 provides examples of each approach.

Within each of the intervention categories listed in Table 9.1, a therapist may use an occupation-focused approach incorporating occupation as the focus of intervention (Fisher, 2014) or an occupation-based approach that uses occupation within the intervention itself. Gillen (2019) identified methods of intervention to include (a) exercise or rote practice, (b) contrived occupation (e.g., stacking cones without a relevant context), (c) therapeutic occupation (direct intervention for impairments in the context of occupation), and (d) adaptive/compensatory approaches to address occupational performance. Gillen contended that OBI approaches are often more effective and reflective of occupational therapy practice than exercise or contrived occupations. There are, however, exceptions. For example, while some people

Table 9.1 Examples of approaches to intervention

Intervention approach	Example
Create/Promote *(Does not assume that illness is present)*	Educating and practicing occupations designed to reduce stress (such as a Mindfulness/Meditation group).
Establish/Restore *(Improving skills or abilities)*	Working with a client to take the public bus system to a store (i.e, teaching community mobility).
Maintain *(Providing supports to maintain current skills or abilities without which there may be a decline in function)*	Using an occupational dance program with older adults to maintain movement patterns for functional mobility.
Modify	Using adaptive garden tools and raised garden beds for a person with rheumatoid arthritis to maintain participation in the occupation of gardening.
Prevent	Setting up a workstation to be ergonomically correct to prevent postural issues or overuse injury.

consider exercise a tedious, rote activity, others may consider it a valued occupation and integral to their lifestyle. Some wellness programs for older adults offer virtual group exercises that can be performed in the home. Even though the client is alone and watching the trainer (and perhaps other group members), the context of the activity is vastly different than repetitive movement alone. The client, context, and occupation must all be considered in providing OBI.

Top-down and Bottom-up Approaches

Chapter 8 defined and discussed differences between top-down and bottom-up approaches to evaluation. Intervention approaches may also be categorized as *top down* or *bottom up*. As previously presented, Trombly (1995) identified top down to include the occupation, meaning, and roles of the client as the initial primary focus, whereas the foundational skills, performance patterns, and activity demands are considered later. She identified the bottom-up approach as focusing "on the deficits of components of function, such as strength, range of motion, balance, and so on, which are believed to be prerequisites to successful occupational performance or functioning" (Trombly, 1995, p. 253). Top-down approaches start from the big picture, which entails understanding the individual's involvement in the occupation. Key occupational priorities are identified, as are the role, purpose, and meaning of the occupation (Ideishi, 2003). Intervention strategies may include incorporation of the actual occupation into the intervention along with work on the client's skills, as well as adaptation of the task. Strategies include plans for assuring the occupation fits the client's skill level and capabilities.

Within the bottom-up approach, occupational activity analysis often occurs along with the component skills of the client. Once underlying deficits or needs are identified (e.g., the client has fatigue, which interferes with job performance), the intervention is targeted to remediate the underlying areas of concern. In this example, the therapist may use strengthening and endurance activities to address the underlying fatigue and improve work tolerance. Underlying physical, cognitive, social, and other component skills are addressed with the goal of enhancing occupational performance.

Although top-down approaches are often referred to as inherently more occupation based, using occupation in the intervention technique, bottom-up strategies are ideally occupation focused to work towards maximizing occupational performance in desired areas. For instance, practicing driving using modifications and safety-oriented behaviors for a person with a spinal cord injury would be an example of a top-down OBI as it incorporates occupation into the intervention with the goal of enhancing performance in a desired occupation (driving). Conversely, working on strengthening of a particular muscle group in the upper extremity to enable independent eating would be a bottom-up occupation-focused approach as long as the goal of mealtime feeding independence was identified as a priority by the client. Therefore, both bottom-up and top-down approaches may be used in occupation-focused and occupation-based intervention. There are inherent strengths in both approaches (Weinstock-Zlotnick & Hinojosa, 2004); therapists often use a combination of the two based on the client, context, and occupational considerations.

In a study of occupational therapists using cognitive rehabilitation, Vas et al. (2021) found that there are benefits to both top-down and bottom-up approaches in therapy. The authors stated that there is continued need to educate therapists about the definition of each, and ways to best use these approaches. Often a combined approach seeking to remediate underlying needs identified in the evaluation along with a functional top-down occupation-based approach is useful in providing complete therapy.

Occupation as a Means and an End

Concepts of occupation-based practice include using meaningful occupation as part of the therapy process. In her 1995 Eleanor Clarke Slagle Lecture, Trombly (1995) proposed that within occupational therapy, occupation may be used both as a means "as the therapeutic change agent to remediate impaired abilities or capacities" (p. 964), or as an end, including the incorporation of important tasks and activities, with the end goal of improving functional performance in a meaningful occupation. According to Trombly, occupation used as means is usually more remedial (bottom up) in focus; while occupation as an end is more adaptive/rehabilitative (top down) or requiring a match of the occupation to the client. An example of occupation as an end would be teaching a client to use modified kitchen utensils for successful completion of cooking. Fleming-Castaldy (2014) notes that both approaches can be useful in therapy.

Although Trombly's discussion of *occupation as an end* did not infer that specific occupations were used in therapy, Gray (1998) expanded on these concepts to suggest that occupation is the goal in both approaches and occupational analysis an important part of determining which approach to use for intervention. Gray also noted that if incorporating meaningful, purposeful occupation within intervention using the occupation as an end approach, then there may be overlap between occupation as a means, and occupation as an end. Thus, while occupation is a core focus of both approaches, in one case occupation is part of a strategy for achieving an outcome and in the other the performance of an occupation is the outcome itself.

Gillen (2019) usefully summarized Trombly's occupation as a means and an end distinction with the following intervention-related descriptors:

Occupation as a Means

- Using occupation as the change agent
- Including interventions such as games, crafts, daily living activities, etc.
- Using more constrained responses as compared to occupation as an end

- Interventions are chosen based on clients' interests and the potential to achieve goals related to an impairment
- Providing a "just right challenge."

Occupation as an End

- Use of occupations that are involved in the direct teaching of a task or the end goal of therapy
- Directly teaching a task
- Using client abilities to learn a task
- Providing task adaptations
- Use of a rehabilitative or skills training approach
- The therapist serves as the teacher or adaptor of the task
- Influenced by information processing theories
- Not necessarily used for making a therapeutic change.

Gillen noted that both occupation as a means and occupation used as an end may be combined therapeutically whereby the therapist uses clinical reasoning skills to determine which parts of therapy would use each approach. Whether using occupation as a means or an end, the practical benefit, meaning, purpose, and perceived value by the client are considered throughout the occupational therapy process.

It is useful to note that, when considering occupation as a means or occupation as an end, the same occupation may be used in both approaches. For example, consider the occupation of artistic painting for leisure. Perhaps a client is working on attention skills and stress reduction and enjoys painting. An occupational therapist may use painting in therapy as a means toward the end goal of improving stress reduction (se Figure 9.1). Conversely, if an individual earned a living through their art and had a traumatic injury that prevented resumption of work, the goal of returning to professional painting would be occupation as an end. Here, the therapeutic modalities used to achieve the end goal may or may not involve painting itself. Thus, occupations may be used in therapy both as a means and as an end.

Perceptions of and Barriers to Occupation-based Intervention

Occupation-based practice uses occupational engagement throughout the occupational therapy process (Tommaso et al., 2016). In using occupation as an agent of change, therapists focus on incorporating meaningful occupation into the intervention process (Fisher, 2014), yet challenges exist in modern day health care settings, particularly with quotas, shorter lengths of stay, and the prevalence of other approaches in practice. Tommaso et al. (2016) conducted a qualitative study

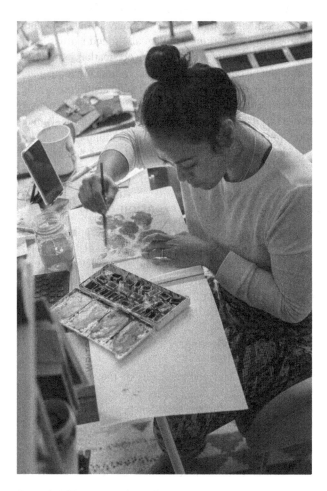

Figure 9.1 The occupation of painting may be used in therapy as a means or an end (photo courtesy of Dushawn Jovic by Unsplash)

of occupational therapists in Australia and found that, although therapists believed occupation-based practice and OBI was important, the focus on impairment-driven intervention was prevalent within the institutional cultures that influenced therapists' practice. The study emphasized the importance of educational programs, including integrated curricula that promote OBI. Mulligan et al. (2014) found similar results in a survey of occupational therapy practitioners in New Hampshire. The investigators found that, while therapists value client-centered occupation-based intervention, more often focus was placed on remediation of performance skills. There were site-specific differences in some settings; for instance, some therapists in hospitals had resource limitations, such as a lack of available space, time, or access to specific assessments and materials. A Malaysian Delphi study with 15 occupational therapists (most working in hospitals) found similar barriers to OBI, including therapists feeling unprepared to use occupation in practice, cultural considerations within the health-care system that promote movement and strength over the use of occupation, difficulties using OBI in an acute care setting, and barriers in the clients themselves not understanding the practical benefit of OBI. To promote greater use of OBI, the authors identified the need for stronger occupation-based education, reflective practice, research, and training.

The following section identifies general guidelines and considerations for OBI.

Guidelines for Occupation-based Intervention (OBI)

The literature reveals varying definitions and views of what occupation-based practice and occupation-based intervention involve. Waehrens et al. (2022) conducted a comprehensive mapping of international scholars to develop a conceptual model of OBI. The resulting model included (a) client factors (e.g., age, gender, motivation), (b) the sociocultural context (cultural background and beliefs, social support, etc.), and (c) structural influences (e.g., sociopolitical influences and organizational culture).

Key practices in OBI included the following:

- Artful use of occupation (skills and competencies of the therapist using occupation in intervention)
- Evidence-based use of occupation (theory, experience, evidence)
- Collaboration to promote occupation (client and therapist)
- Coordinating intervention fit (fit between client and intervention)
- Considering client factors (physical, cognitive and emotional status)
- Awareness of client's sociocultural context (culture, environment, family, social support, etc.)
- Addressing structural influences influencing the use of occupation (this could include systems related factors involving delivery systems, or organizations, etc.)

The conceptual map facilitates understanding of factors influencing the use of occupation as a change agent in OBI. Occupational therapists must holistically consider all factors when working with the client to determine the best approach to intervention.

Although concepts of meaning weren't explicitly stated in Waehrens' (2022) conceptual map, they may be inferred in the broad range of client-related factors related to occupational engagement. Psillas and Stav (2021) conducted a grounded theory study to develop a dynamic model of occupation-based practice. Key constructs they identified included (a) authentic occupation, (b) engaged occupation, (c) meaningful and purposeful value, and (d) therapeutic intent. The authors contend that actual participation in meaningful occupation is most closely aligned with occupation-based practice and that there must be purposeful use of the occupation with a specific rationale and therapeutic intent (see Figure 9.2). Thus, the mere use of an occupation without a client-relevant reason would not constitute OBI. For instance, if a client with a hip replacement loved knitting, its use would not be considered therapeutic unless it connected to an appropriate goal for intervention (e.g., developing coping skills rather than rehab of the hip). Similar to literature previously discussed, the authors acknowledge factors that may affect the therapist's ability to practice OBI, such as physical space, institutional policies, and client factors. Therapists must use clinical reasoning skills to determine how best to implement OBI.

To facilitate meaningful occupation, the therapist incorporates previous concepts discussed, including the client factors and narrative, the assessment of occupation, and application of theoretical frameworks considering the impact of the environment and context on occupation. Peterson and Stoffel (2022) applied concepts of recovery to the facilitation of occupation. Table 9.2 provides examples of model-based reasoning that may be used in the occupational therapy process to facilitate occupational engagement in clients based on their work.

In addition to the incorporation of meaningful occupation in OBI, Ikiugu et al. (2016, 2018) studied concepts of meaningful or psychologically rewarding occupations. The authors found that while both meaningful and psychologically rewarding occupations were engaging, meaningful activities were often

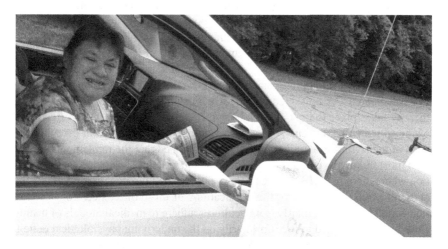

Figure 9.2 This individual enjoys delivering papers for her work, it is an important part of her occupation-based intervention (photo courtesy of Kristine Haertl).

Table 9.2 Facilitating occupation

Client's personal narrative	Client's occupations	Occupation-based models (e.g., PEO, PEOP, CMOP)
Reason for referral to OT	Occupational history & roles	Explore environmental supports and barriers— develop strategies
Identify what occupations are supported or hindered due to present condition.	Assessments of roles, habits, routines, and occupational performance	Assess community connectedness and available resources
Education on diagnosis or condition	Education on meaning and occupation	Planning and problem solving for community integration
Identify how condition impacts daily occupation	Occupational analysis and personal reflection	Occupation-based model (e.g., PEO, PEOP, CMOP)
Education on strategies for occupational engagement	Prioritize current and future occupations to address in therapy	Explore environmental supports and barriers— develop strategies

Adapted from Peterson & Stoffel (2022).

mentally stimulating, while those incorporating fun were perceived as psychologically rewarding. In addition, psychologically rewarding occupations often led to the experience of flow, described as a state of involvement in an activity where perceived time is suspended and a heightened sense of personal satisfaction in the activity results (Csikszentmihalyi, 1997). The authors concluded that occupational therapists should include both meaningful and psychologically rewarding occupational experiences within therapy.

A final consideration in the implementation of OBI is that in addition to the setting and context, client factors, and perceptions, it is important to note that the therapist's views, training, and culture may all affect the level to which OBI is implemented. As presented earlier, it is not only the environment in which therapy takes place (e.g., a client's hospital room in acute care) that affects the extent to which OBI occurs, but also the cultural views and health care models used in the setting. Kaunnil et al. (2021) maintained that the implementation of OBI must fit into the cultural values, beliefs, and practices customary to the location where therapy is provided. Chapter 5 discussed differences in individualistic and collectivist societies and the implications of those differences for occupation-based practice. Similarly, some cultures adhere to medical models of health care practice designed to focus primarily on the underlying physiological deficit (e.g., lack of mobility in a joint). Yet within such cultural and societal settings, the focus in occupational therapy should continue to emphasize either the use of occupation as a therapeutic means, or the use of therapy techniques designed to enhance meaningful performance. Continued research is needed to explore ways to implement occupation-based practice in various cultures (Kaunnil et al., 2021).

BOX 9.1 OCCUPATION IN ACTION: INTERVENTION— NEONATAL INTENSIVE CARE UNIT

Within the technical and fast-paced Neonatal Intensive Care Unit (NICU) environment, occupational therapists are uniquely poised to facilitate the occupational performance of infants, parents/caregivers, and the infant–parent dyad. In a high-acuity medical setting where specialized professionals rely heavily on objective, quantifiable measures of infant growth, stability, and health, occupational therapists are routinely challenged to embrace non-reductionistic thinking and approach intervention from an occupation-centered and relationship-based perspective. As a certified neonatal therapist, the author of the following case example receives frequent referrals for feeding evaluation and treatment. For medically fragile or premature infants, bottle-feeding and breastfeeding can be extremely difficult. Layers of complexity must be peeled away to reveal the barriers and enablers of occupational performance. It is in this moment of task-level analysis that occupational therapists can stretch beyond development of a plan that may (very appropriately) address the inner mechanisms of the infant to one that powerfully shifts the dialogue surrounding feeding skill in the NICU. More than administering oral-motor coordination or suck strength intervention, there is an opportunity for occupational therapists to offer transformational co-occupational *mealtime* intervention.

Case Example

Sophie was born 11 weeks early and weighed roughly 3 pounds (1.4 kg). Though still premature, she is now five weeks old and stable enough to begin feeding by mouth. She has been diagnosed with bronchopulmonary dysplasia, which affects her breathing rate, oxygen levels, and endurance when participating in her daily occupations. Sophie's mother, Anna, wanted to breastfeed but stopped pumping breastmilk due to a medication change; therefore, she plans to bottle-feed Sophie. Sophie has been referred to occupational therapy for feeding evaluation and treatment.

After reviewing Sophie's medical chart, the author called Anna to schedule a time for the feeding evaluation. In the NICU, staff recognize and honor how important it is for parents to be present for any "firsts." As this was Sophie's first bottle-feeding, Anna's availability was arranged. In speaking to Anna and gathering her narrative, it was reasoned that Anna was primarily concerned with eliminating her infant's barriers to feeding and that she wished to receive education on how to keep Sophie safe from choking during the feeding. Based on these narrative insights and Anna's stated goals, the PEOP model was chosen as a suitable approach to develop the intervention plan. During a feeding session later that evening, Anna responded well to the therapist's *Therapeutic Use of Self* and some appropriate education and training. The infant responded well to preparatory methods that included sucking on a pacifier and being swaddled before bottle-feeding began. Anna worked with the therapist to create a low-stimulation environment for mealtime by dimming the overhead lights and speaking to Sophie in a soft voice. Additionally, choking was prevented by using a slow-flow nipple on Anna's bottle of choice. To foster infant–mother attachment and socialization as part of the mealtime plan, ways to position Sophie during feeding were discussed.

Rather than medicalizing the feeding session in her treatment note (e.g., "The patient ingested 75% of the prescribed volume over 20 minutes using a slow-flow bottle"), occupational therapists can provide humanized occupational intervention by situating the feeding event within the rich context and pattern of *mealtime* (e.g., "Sophie's mom held her in the cradled position during bottle-feeding. Sophie used a slow-flow bottle to increase feeding coordination and preserve energy to visually engage with mom. Sophie finished 75% of her bottle without signs of stress or discomfort. Mom held Sophie and talked to her while the rest of her feeding was given through her feeding tube").

Application Questions

1. Who is (are) the occupational therapist's client(s) in this case example?
2. What concepts of co-occupation are demonstrated?
3. Beyond the bottle-feeding activity, what other aspects of *mealtime* could be considered by occupational therapists in this case example?

(Ashlea D. Cardin, OTD, OTR/L, BCP, CNT)

Service Delivery Models

Although occupation-focused and occupation-based intervention are often referred to in relation to an individual client or patient, service delivery may be expanded to include families and caregivers (e.g., in pediatrics or populations

Table 9.3 Selected examples of client occupational therapy outcomes

Client	Outcome
76-year-old man with recent stroke	Increased independence in dressing
Three-year-old girl with cerebral palsy	Facilitation of co-play between parent and child
Group home serving persons with intellectual and developmental disabilities (IDD).	Re-design of space to facilitate socialization and occupational participation
Young woman with eating disorder	Improved understanding of nutrition, improved ability to plan meals and shop for groceries.

with dementia), groups (e.g., in a mental health occupation-based group in a psychiatric facility), or with populations and systems (e.g., consultation with a residential service provider for persons with intellectual and developmental disabilities). Intervention should continue to focus on the client/stakeholder factors, the context in which service delivery takes place, and consideration of occupation-based outcomes. Table 9.3 gives some examples of desired outcomes for various **service delivery models**.

Although each of the above examples represents a different service delivery model, in each case the methods of intervention would be considered occupation-focused or occupation-based.

The therapist uses clinical reasoning to determine the focus of intervention. For instance, if a therapist working in a psychiatric hospital is facilitating a higher-level living skills group, methods used for teaching cooking skills would likely not only include the discussion of safety and nutrition considerations, but also actual practice of the cooking skill. In a situation of working with clients who will return to an independent or semi-independent living situation and enjoy cooking, the therapeutic goal of teaching safe cooking is in line with expected client outcomes. Conversely, if working with individuals who have challenged cognition and severe psychosis, the use of cooking in a task group may be an OBI used for socialization and other therapeutic effects, yet may not have the primary goal of teaching safe cooking skills. This consideration would be relevant if the client was expected to move to a supported living situation or group home in which meal preparation is completed by staff. To summarize, the reason for referral to occupational therapy, the meaning of the occupation to the client, and priorities of therapy may all affect the service delivery and methods used for intervention.

Therapeutic Use of Self

A final consideration related to OBI includes the role of the therapist and relationship with the client. Therapeutic use of self refers to "the therapist's role in working consciously with the interpersonal side of the therapeutic relationship to facilitate an optimal experience and outcome for the client" (Solman & Clouston, 2016, p. 514). The development of rapport and ability to engage with the client in the therapeutic process is integral to the outcome of therapy. Taylor et al. (2009) found that while occupational therapy practitioners value therapeutic use of self as an important part of the therapy process, a comprehensive survey indicated that most therapists felt unprepared in this area and that more training and education is needed. With respect to education on the client–practitioner relationship, Taylor (2008) developed the Intentional Relationship Model (IRM) which identifies interactive styles used to relate to clients. The University of Illinois Chicago (2022) identified ten principles of IRM:

1. Critical self-awareness is essential in the intentional use of self
2. Interpersonal self-discipline is fundamental to the effective use of self
3. It is necessary to keep the head before the heart (therapeutic goals are paramount in client relationships)
4. Mindful empathy is required to know the client
5. Importance of developing one's interpersonal knowledge base
6. A range of therapeutic modes can be used interchangeably in OT provided they are flexibly and purely applied
7. The client defines a successful relationship
8. Activity focus must be balanced with interpersonal focus
9. Application of IRM must be informed by OT core values and ethics
10. Cultural competency is central to practice.

The above principles highlight the importance of educating oneself not only concerning occupation-based intervention strategies, but also on the development of core therapeutic skills in the client–practitioner relationship.

Carol Davis, a physical therapist, has devoted much of her career to the development of exercises and activities designed to help students and practitioners enhance their self-awareness and communication skills for therapy (Davis & Musolino, 2016). Davis emphasizes the importance of coming to know oneself in the therapeutic relationship and developing skills through self-reflective activities and interactive experiences with other practitioners aimed at understanding the dynamics central to the therapeutic relationship. This approach is also designed to teach faculty how to educate on the intentional use of self in the therapeutic relationship.

As therapists consider the use of self in practice, a key focus includes the client perspective. Haertl (2017) emphasized the importance of multiple ways of knowing in the therapeutic use of self. Intentional use of self involves not only knowledge of the concepts, but also acknowledgment of how intuition, emotion, imagination, and other mental processes facilitate the understanding and development of empathy for the client's perspective. The therapist should acknowledge the differences in worldview, beliefs, and perspectives that may exist between the client and therapist and learn to build rapport and facilitate the therapeutic relationship with awareness of these differences. For instance, Box 9.2 describes special considerations in providing occupational therapy services to the Amish community. A therapist must not only apply principles of cultural humility and cultural understanding, but also consider how to best develop rapport and nurture the therapist–client relationship in working with clients from this population.

BOX 9.2 OCCUPATION IN ACTION: OLD ORDER AMISH INTERVENTION

One of the most enjoyable aspects of occupational therapy is the challenge to respond creatively to the needs of pediatric clients and their families. Creativity flourishes when people, life events, and materials intersect, and occupational therapists are beautifully positioned to help translate the child and family's creative capacity into purposeful occupational participation. As a *pro bono* therapist within an Old Order Amish community, I have learned that creativity and ingenuity abound in the most unexpected places—from the field where oat shocks are intricately stacked and sculpted to keep the seeds dry, to the barn where children use homemade sizing boxes to sort tomatoes or eggs, or to the home where an infant's wooden highchair magically folds into a child's rocking horse by simply repositioning a few latches, pegs, and straps. While each of these clever examples is unique in its form and function, they inherently share a characteristic of ingenuity valued by the Amish: Purpose. Recognizing purpose as a culturally meaningful attribute of creativity, occupational therapy practitioners can either deploy creativity as a response to problem solving or, more collaboratively, invite their clients' creativity, resourcefulness, or inventiveness into the intervention spaces to maximize occupational performance.

Case Example

Amanda is a 21-year-old mother and Amish community member. Due to pregnancy complications, she recently delivered her second child in hospital instead of at home surrounded by her large family. The baby has been admitted to the Neonatal Intensive Care Unit (NICU), where only Amanda and her husband, Sam, may stay at the bedside. Amanda's primary support system (her parents, grandparents, and older sisters) were not allowed to visit the hospital due to the risks of COVID-19 and the impending flu season.

The therapist received an occupational therapy order to help Amanda prepare for future breastfeeding. Amanda reported that her breastmilk supply had "dropped way off" due to high stress levels, eating only hospital food, and her dislike of using the electric breast pumps at the bedside. She lamented that if she were home, she would be able to hold the baby when she wanted, practice putting the baby to breast, and use a piston-style hand pump to help "build up" her breastmilk supply. She added that "it's hard for us to get our minds off of [her milk supply] because we're not keeping busy … we're doing a lot of watching and waiting." Sam, a furniture builder, added that he was used to working all day in his shop, and being "cooped up" in the hospital only increased his worry about the baby's nutrition. After gathering the family's narrative, the therapist asked about which breastfeeding goal they would like to address first. Both expressed disappointment that only electric breast pumps were available (they preferred simplicity over technology) and wanted to use their familiar piston-style single hand pumps to extract milk. Amanda noted that using the hospital's pump to extract milk from both breasts at the same time was helpful in increasing her milk supply. Having learned that Sam was talented in creating functional pieces of furniture, the therapist asked him the following question: "If you could design a dual-sided breast pump for Amanda, what would it look like?" The reasoning behind posing this question extended beyond curiosity or friendly conversation—it was aimed at determining how creative theory, occupational behavior, self-determination, and a strengths-based perspective could be used to support the family's well-being and occupational performance goals. Immediately, a smile appeared and widened across Sam's face. He stood up, retrieved a piece of paper, and began sketching with Amanda's input. That evening, I checked back with Sam and Amanda, who said the day had passed quickly for them. Sam excitedly showed me a rough blueprint for a wooden treadle-style breast pump, one that mirrored the mechanism of Amanda's foot-operated sewing machine at home. When Amanda pushed on the foot treadle, a belt would move a piece of wood that was attached to two hand-pump pistons, thus extracting milk from both breasts at the same time. Sam planned to make a "lightweight" version of his breast pump on his next visit home. He requested that the therapist seek permission for him to bring his device into the NICU for Amanda's use. The therapist's advocacy succeeded, and permission was granted.

Application Questions

1. In this case example, breastfeeding was considered a subgoal within a larger occupational priority. What overarching goal might Sam and Amanda be working toward?

2. In what ways did the occupational therapist use her creative capacity to help empower and build self-advocacy in the family?

(Ashlea D. Cardin, OTD, OTR/L, BCP, CNT)

Conclusion

Occupation-focused and occupation-based practice are fundamental to occupational therapy. Interventions of this nature are evidence based, client centered, use professional reasoning skills, and are facilitated through the therapist–client relationship. Intervention techniques using occupation may be top down or bottom up and may use occupation as either a means toward a therapeutic goal or as the performance-related goal of therapy. Occupation-based service delivery may occur with individuals, groups, and populations and is designed to promote health through occupational engagement.

BOX 9.3 THE POINT IS:

- Occupation-focused and occupation-based interventions may use top-down or bottom-up approaches to intervention.
- Occupation-based practice incorporates occupation as a means of intervention; the occupations selected should be meaningful to the client.
- Occupation-focused and occupation-based interventions may be implemented in a variety of service delivery methods (e.g., individuals, families, and groups).
- In addition to client factors, contextual factors related to the anticipated living environment are relevant to the selection of intervention methods.

Acknowledgment

The authors thank Dr. Ashlea Cardin for her valued contributions to the completion of this chapter.

References

American Occupational Therapy Association (AOTA). (2020). Occupational therapy practice framework: Domain and process (4th ed.). *American Journal of Occupational Therapy, 74*(Suppl. 2), 7412410010. https://doi.org/10.5014/ajot.2020.74S2001

Backman, C. L., Christiansen, C. H., Hooper, B. R., Pierce, D., & Price, M. P. (2021).Occupational science concepts essential to occupation-based practice: Development of expert consensus. *The American Journal of Occupational Therapy, 75*(6), 7506205120. https://doi.org/10.5014/ajot.2021.049090

Csikszentmihalyi, M. (1997). *Finding flow: The psychology of engagement with everyday life.* Basic Books.

Davis, C. M., & Musolino, G. M. (2016). *Patient practitioner interaction: An experiential manual for developing the art of health care* (6th ed.). Slack.

Fisher, A. G. (2014). Occupation-centred, occupation-based, occupation-focused: Same, same or different? *Scandinavian Journal of Occupational Therapy, 21*, 96–107. https://doi.org/10.3109/11038128.2014.952912

Fleming-Castaldy, R. (2014). Part II. Theoretical and conceptual frameworks to guide occupation-based practice. In R. Fleming-Castaldy (Ed.), *Perspectives for occupation-based practice: Foundations and future of occupational therapy* (3rd ed., pp. 109–114). AOTA Press.

Gallagher, M., Muldoon, O. T., & Pettigrew, J. (2015). An integrative review of social and occupational factors influencing health and wellbeing. *Frontiers in Psychology, 6*(1281), 1–11. https://doi.org/10.3389/fpsyg .2015.01281

Gillen, G. (2019). Occupational therapy interventions for individuals. In B. A. Schell & G. Gillen (Eds.), *Willard & Spackman's occupational therapy* (13th ed., pp. 413–435). Wolters Kluwer.

Gray, J. M. (1998). Putting occupation into practice: Occupation as ends, occupation as means. *American Journal of Occupation Therapy, 52*, 354–364. https://doi.org/10 .5014/ajot.52.5.354

Haertl, K. (2017). *Therapeutic use of self and the power of occupation: Dancing to the beat of the music.* Occupationaltherapy.com articles

Ideishi, R. (2003). Occupational adaptation: Influence of occupation on assessment and treatment. In P. Kramer,J. Hinojosa, & C. B. Royeen (Eds.), *Perspectives in human occupation: Participation in life* (pp. 278–296). Lippincott Williams & Wilkins.

Ikiugu, M. N., Hoyme, A. K., Mueller, B., & Reinke, R. (2016). Difference between meaningful and psychologically rewarding occupations: Findings from two pilot studies. *Journal of Occupational Science, 23*(2), 266–277. https://doi.org/10.1080 /14427 591.2015.10854 31.

Ikiugu, M. N., Lucas-Molitor, W., Feldhacker, D., Gebhart, C., Spier, M., Kapels, L., Arnold, R., & Gaikowski, R. (2018). Guidelines for occupational therapy interventions based on meaningful and psychologically rewarding occupations. *Journal of Happiness Studies, 20*, 2027–2053. https://doi.org/10.1007/s10902-018 -0030-z

Kaunnil, A., Khemthong, S., Sriphetcharawut, S., Thichanpiang, P., Sansri, V., Thongchoomsin, S., Permpoonputtana, K., & Smith, C. R. (2021). Occupational therapists' experiences and perspectives towards occupation-based practice in

Thailand: A mixed-methods study. *British Journal of Occupational Therapy*, *84*(1), 54–64. https://doi.org/10.1177/0308022620910402

Mulligan, S., Prudhomme White, B., & Arthanat, S. (2014). An examination of occupation-based, client-centered, evidence-based occupational therapy practices in New Hampshire. *OTJR: Occupation, Participation and Health*, *34*(2), 106–116. https://doi.org/10.3928/15394492-20140226-01

Occupational Therapy Australia (2018). *Evidence-based practice position statement.* https://otaus.com.au/publicassets/90977488-f433-e911-a2c2b75c2fd918c5/ebpposi tionstatement.pdf

Petersen, E., & Stoffel, V. (2022) *Occupational discovery for recovery: How occupational therapy aligns with the recovery model to support engagement in meaningful occupations.* American Occupational Therapy Association Specialty Conference. Columbus, Ohio.

Psillas, S. M., & Stav, W. B. (2021). Development of the dynamic model of occupation-based practice. *Open Journal of Occupational Therapy*, *9*(4), 1–14. https://doi.org/10 .15453/2168-6408.1807

Solman, B., & Clouston, C. (2016). Occupational therapy and therapeutic use of self. *British Journal of Occupational Therapy*, *79*(8), 514–516.

Taylor, R. R. (2008). *The intentional relationship: Occupational therapy and use of self.* F.A. Davis.

Taylor, R. R., Lee, S. W., Kielhofner, G., & Ketkar, M. (2009). Therapeutic use of self: A nationwide survey of practitioners' attitudes and experiences. *American Journal of Occupational Therapy*, *63*(2), 198–207. https://doi.org/10.5014/ajot.63.2.198

Tommaso, A. D., Isbel, S., Scarvell, J., & Wicks, A. (2016). Occupational therapists' perceptions of occupation in practice: An exploratory study. *Australian Occupational Therapy Journal*, *63*, 206–213. https://doi.org/10.1111/1440-1630.12289

Trombly, C. A. (1995). Occupation: Purposefulness and meaningfulness as therapeutic mechanisms. 1995 Elanor Clarke Slagle Lecture. *American Journal of Occupational Therapy*, *49*, 960–972. https://doi.org/10.5014/ajot.49.10.960

University of Illinois Chicago. (2022). *About IRM.* https://irm.ahs.uic.edu/about-irm/#:~ :text=The%20Intentional%20Relationship%20Model%20describes,productive %20relationship%20with%20a%20client

Vas, A. K., Luedke, A., Ortiz, E., & Neville, M. (2021). Bottom-up and top-down cognitive rehabilitation following traumatic brain injury—Occupational therapists perspective: An online survey study. *The Indian Journal of Occupational Therapy*, *53*, 56–63. https://doi.org/10.4103/ijoth.ijoth_8_21

Waehrens, E. E., Nielson, K. T., Cutchin, M., Fritz, H., Jonsson, H., & la Cour, K. (2022). Fostering change through occupation-based intervention: An international joint group concept mapping study. *OTJR: Occupation, Participation and Health*, *42*(1), 10–21. https://journals.sagepub.com/doi/10.1177/15394492211038283

Weinstock-Zlotnick, G., & Hinojosa, J. (2004). Bottom-up or top-down evaluation: Is one better than the other? *American Journal of Occupational Therapy*, *58*, 594–599. https://doi.org/10.4103/ijoth.ijoth_8_21

Chapter 10

Human Occupation and the Future

Introduction

The observation that the world is changing rapidly seems obvious. The first two decades of this century have witnessed a global pandemic, multiple extreme weather events, global terrorism, regional ideological violence and conflict, and social and political unrest. Extraordinary events are commonplace, and one wonders if changes are happening so quickly and frequently that the concept of "normal" is now outdated and meaningless. The goal of this chapter is to describe how these changes may likely influence human occupation in the remainder of the 21st century. In the following sections, major categories of change will be discussed.

The Digital Tsunami

It is hard to imagine a world without smartphones, the Internet, virtual conferencing, and feedback loops. Yet over four decades ago author John Naisbett (1982), a writer and futures expert, wrote a popular book called *Megatrends*, forecasting ten major changes of global importance. Naisbett's book sold millions of copies and had a remarkable impact on social conversation. He correctly predicted America's transformation from a postindustrial society to an information society; and forecast important related trends such as networking, decentralized decision making, the rise of the global economy and greater societal demands for personal choice. But Naisbett's predictions occurred before the invention of the Internet and thus he vastly underestimated the impact of information technology. Futures scientists examine trends and make forecasts based on what *has* occurred. But they cannot predict *black swan events*. These are irregular, unexpected occurrences that can have transformative consequences. Examples include the dramatic rise of the Internet, the 9/11 terrorist attack, the war in Ukraine, and numerous natural disasters including hurricanes, floods, and earthquakes.

DOI: 10.4324/9781003242185-10

The Internet and Digital Connectivity

At the time of its invention, the Internet was perhaps the most transformative lifestyle technology ever developed as the following statistics illustrate. According to Internet lifestats.com (2023), in 1993 there were 130 websites in the world and just over 14 million Internet users. Now, there are over 1 billion websites and around 5 billion Internet users (Petrosyan, 2023). These users spend, *on average,* three hours daily on the Internet, but nearly eight hours connected to digital technologies (Statista, 2023). Nearly one-third of the U.S. population reports using the Internet almost constantly, with 44% of adults aged 18–50 in that category (Pew Research Center, 2021). However, 7% of the U.S. population reports *never* using the Internet, and this category represents 25% of persons over 65. The demographic category with the most Internet users is adults aged 25–34.

Kuntsman & Miyake (2019) suggest that existing views of technology should be reconsidered to acknowledge how the growing interconnectivity of digital technologies is creating environments and habitats that make it difficult to live without digital connectivity. Those whose economic circumstances limit digital access will likely become more culturally isolated and disadvantaged, while better educated and affluent people will become more connected, but also more susceptible to its adverse consequences.

Health Consequences of Excessive Internet Use

Most social scientists agree that current levels of Internet use have adverse consequences and constitute a threat to public health for all ages (Neophytou et al., 2019; Young, 2015). Excessive screen time by young children is of special concern because it is influenced by their parents and may thwart developmental progress (Madigan, et al., 2019). Excessive Internet use in preschool children is related to attention deficits and other symptoms resembling autism-spectrum disorders (Heffler et al., 2020; Tamana et al., 2019). These data are concerning, given that Internet use can easily become habitually compulsive.

Compulsive Internet use was first studied in 1996 and rapidly gained interest among mental health professionals as a type of addiction (Vadivu & Chupradit, 2020). Now recognized as a global problem, the DSM-V (APA, 2013) and the ICD-11 now include descriptions for **Internet Gaming Disorder (IGM)**, considered a specialized type of **Internet addiction.**

Time use scientists who have studied the displacement of other activities by the Internet are most concerned about its impact on sleep. Not only has the amount of sleep by Internet users declined, the quality of sleep has also been affected by exposure to the bright light of digital screens. Not surprisingly, disturbed sleep as well as insomnia are consequences of habitual or excessive Internet use (Dissing et al., 2022; Dresp-Langley & Hutt, 2022).

In addition to sleep problems, heavy Internet use can disrupt relationships and jeopardize employment through disruption of a person's ability to manage time, energy, and attention. An important part of Internet addiction therapy is helping addicts recognize their rationalizations and acknowledge excessive gaming or social media use as a type of escapism. Internet use addiction is a habit disorder, which restricts time available for participating in important health-related activities such as social relationships, productive work, and self-care. Excessive digital use may benefit from intervention by occupational therapists working in mental health, especially those with experience in lifestyle problems and those qualified to provide cognitive behavioral therapy for internet addiction (CBT-IA) (Eakman et al., 2017).

Excessive Internet use can also have other mental health consequences. Ivie et al. (2020) reported a **meta-analysis** of studies reporting an association between social media use and depression in adolescents. Vidal and colleagues (2020) corroborated this trend and noted the association between excessive social media use and suicide in adolescent women. Studies have shown that reducing social media use among adolescents results in improved measures of well-being, suggesting that this age group is susceptible to harmful emotional consequences of social media (Haidt & Allen, 2020).

Lifestyle Changes from Virtual Environments

The mandated social isolation of the pandemic of 2020 created circumstances where many people became unemployed, were forced to shutter small businesses, or were required to work or study online. The widespread use of virtual meeting platforms such as Zoom led to advanced capabilities to facilitate meetings (such as breakout sessions and polling). Advanced meeting platforms can be improved by **virtual reality** (VR), **augmented reality** (AR), and **artificial intelligence** (AI) (Diplomacy.edu, 2020). For example, the use of hybrid meetings assisted by virtual assistants to schedule, connect, monitor, and document meetings is anticipated (Diplomacy.edu, 2020). These rapidly evolving changes will affect how work is organized, who does it, and the status of those who participate (Tan et al., 2021).

It is widely agreed that pandemic restrictions disrupted daily routines and afforded "down time" for reflection, influencing the way many people viewed paid work (Peters et al., 2022). The flexibility of working from home, freedom from long commutes, and a reconsideration of personal priorities fostered consideration of employment alternatives. In many cases, this resulted in creative freelancing, using the Internet in an opportunistic way for home employment, characterized by short-term contracts rather than traditional long-term office-based work. This transformation gave further impetus to the **gig economy**, since some people decided to continue home-based work rather than resume their traditional commuting jobs after the mandatory lockdowns (e.g., Cheng, 2021).

However, although recent studies have shown an increase in online freelance work, the *actual* impact on the workforce and economy over the past two decades has been less than 3% (Collins et al., 2019).

More importantly, the pandemic influenced fundamental worker attitudes toward workplace expectations. Employers were pressured into relaxing policies related to working from home (Smite et al., 2023). Although some changes were already under way, the pandemic forced retail sales, health care delivery, real estate, investment, architecture, and commercial art to hasten creative and effective online alternatives to traditional modes of service delivery (Kane et al., 2021). Many of those innovations have continued.

Digital advances are also changing the production and manufacture of raw materials and goods, as well as inspiring innovations in knowledge sharing. These changes are significant enough to label them a **Fourth Industrial Revolution** (Schwab, 2017; see Table 10.1). The basic impetus behind this global change is artificial intelligence and its applications in **automation** and **robotics**.

Artificial Intelligence, Automation, and Robotics

Automated machines or devices that use digital technologies and artificial intelligence are having a disruptive effect on society as robotic technologies evolve. A *robot* can be defined as any automated machine that can sense, compute, and act (IEEE, 2022). There are no robots without artificial intelligence (AI), since AI implies the ability of a machine to mimic human behavior and use knowledge, at least at a rudimentary level. Three types of robotic technologies mentioned in this chapter include **robots, bots,** and **chatbots**.

Robots do their work through a physical interface or presence, such as those found on assembly lines. Unfortunately, many people still think of robots as futuristic mechanical humans, but the technology behind these sci-fi visions of interactive human replicas is still in its relative infancy. For years, industry has been using robots for a host of applications, such as in **3D printing** and fabrication of sophisticated high precision tools, products, and devices in every industry, including defense, the food industry, pharmaceuticals, and medicine (Dupont et al., 2021). New applications are under development continuously (Shahrubudin et al., 2019).

Bots are complex computer programs that accurately perform routine or repetitive tasks. They can search, identify, sort, calculate, and route based on complex algorithms. Bots are considered back-end technologies—they are behind such functions as identity recognition and targeted marketing. They are also used for malicious purposes in malware.

Finally, *chatbots* are a specialized type of bot that interacts with human users through simulated conversation. They have programmed responses based on the identification of phrases provided by users using natural language processing.

Table 10.1 A history of global industrial revolutions

Period		Transformative development(s)	Societal impacts
I	1740s–1860s	The invention of steam power and its application in work, manufacturing, and transportation.	Dramatically improved worker productivity and improved work efficiency in industry and agriculture, improving wages and standard of living. Revolutionary changes in transportation through locomotives, railways, and steamboats.
II	1870s–1914	The invention of electricity, the telephone, and better scientific instruments leading to innovations driven by science in chemistry, metallurgy, food production, refrigeration, food preparation and transport, explosives, and medical knowledge.	Advances led to rapid standardization and industrialization. The growth of usable and practical knowledge from scientific understanding enabled important and rapid changes in medicine, the quality of goods, medical care, and working conditions. It also led to urbanization, migration, and the creation and use of destructive weapons.
III	1950s–early 2000s	The invention of semiconductors, personal computers and the Internet led to the rise of automation and the transformation from analog to digital devices.	This period is sometimes called the automation revolution. Many processes became semi-automatic or automatic. The Internet and digital devices transformed information sharing and communication. Renewable energy sources (wind, solar etc.) were developed.
IV	2000–?	Advancements in digital computing with higher speed and memory enabling wider Internet use, developments in artificial intelligence and their application in robotics and the connectivity of the Internet of Things (IoT).	Changes in work by increasing convenience and efficiency; continued increases in use and reliance on the Internet for social interaction, commerce, and information sharing. Development and wider use of drones, autonomous vehicles, and robotics. Emergence of generative artificial intelligence in chatbots.

Future industrial revolutions based on transformative technologies

Based on Groumpos (2021). Creative commons open access.

Generative Artificial Intelligence

Transformational AI systems have now evolved called **generative artificial intelligence**. These chatbot AI systems require vast amounts of data, ultra-fast computing, and high-level software engineering expertise. Capable of quickly processing vast amounts of text-based information using deep learning algorithms, these systems create new content that equals or surpasses that produced by humans. This content can include audio, software code, images, text, simulations, and videos (Raj & Seamans, 2019). It is widely agreed that enterprises like literature, art, journalism, photography, videography, graphic and web design (and even software coding) will be transformed. Accurately predicting the implications of these disruptive technologies depends on how they are used, and the ethical and moral principles of its builders and users.

Internet of Things (IoT)

In addition to generative AI, another potentially transformative application of AI is the evolving technology of the **Internet of Things** (IoT). This is the basis for smart homes and connects robots designed to perform dedicated tasks ranging from vacuuming floors to controlling temperature and lighting. Of course, use outside the home, especially in industry, is already well under way as an important element of Industry 4.0 (Zeng et al., 2023.

Industries are using IoT and robots to integrate systems, manage resources, and optimize supply chains for optimal efficiency (Raj & Seamans, 2019; Alaa et al., 2017). The transportation industry has applied the IoT to enhance safety and efficiency. Moreover, the development of autonomous vehicles for air, sea, and ground transportation has steadily proceeded (Parekh et al., 2022; see Figure 10.1). Personal transportation has benefitted from shared ride innovations such as Uber™, Lyft™, and Zipcar™, as well as peer-to-peer car rental innovations like Getaround ™, Maven ™, and Turo™. However, for personal transportation, the use of fully autonomous vehicles has been slower because of infrastructure limitations, affordability, and consumer hesitancy (McLeay et al., 2022). Forecasters predict that *shared* autonomous vehicle services represent the most likely scenario affecting the personal use of autonomous cars in the near term (Narayanan et al., 2020).

In medicine and health care, AI and the IoT have permitted greater use of wearable sensors to monitor patient status and analyze data to optimize and personalize care (Khan et al., 2021). There has also been limited development of personal assistants to serve as companions, help manage daily tasks, and provide therapeutic assistance (Martinez-Martin & del Pobil, 2018).

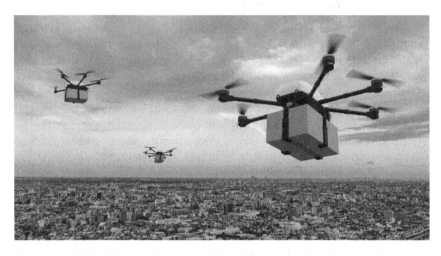

Figure 10.1 AI controlled Autonomous Aerial Vehicles (cargo drones) to speed delivery are in late-stage development (Metamorworks via iStock, used under license)

Workforce Changes Due to Artificial Intelligence and Robotics

Predictions on the displacement of jobs by robotics tend to be overstated, but current estimates suggest that, by 2030, 8% of *manufacturing* jobs globally will have been affected (Oxford Economics, 2019). This does not suggest a net loss of jobs, but it does portend changes in the *types* of work that will be required. These effects will vary regionally based on workforce characteristics, and the types of industry in each location. In the United States, studies suggest that robot deployment reduces jobs at a rate of 1:6 and, where deployed, robots have a modest (<1%) negative impact on wages overall (Acemoglu & Restrepo, 2020). The use of AI will dramatically increase in the years ahead because of the positive economic effects of adopting these new technologies (Graetz & Michaels, 2017), and because, as Harari (2018) described it, AI has two features that humans cannot replicate: *Unlimited networking* and *instant updating*. The current limitations of AI must also be acknowledged and addressed. Humans have an important ability that AI does not: *Intuition*. In the face of uncertainty, the subconscious processing of the human mind informs and enables decision making. When errors result in contexts where humans are working with AI, where should accountability reside? Moreover, what are the potential health and safety consequences for robotics with human–machine interfaces? Howard (2019) noted that the widespread implementation of AI requires improved understanding of worker health implications and less ambiguity concerning accountability.

Job Creation Related to Artificial Intelligence

Aly (2020) points out that, as a disruptive technology, the incorporation of AI into industries takes time. In developing nations, the economic impacts are positive, as product and services motivate increased digital connectivity and stimulate demand. In developed nations, increased efficiencies result in stronger balance sheets, creating investment and expansion. It is likely that the effects on the workforce will be variable over time. Forecasters are reluctant to predict the impact of these changes on vulnerable populations, but new jobs will be created.

For example, skilled and specialized robotics engineers will be required for manufacturing and software and hardware maintenance; and skilled programmers with knowledge of neural network or pattern recognition algorithms and **big data** analytics will be in demand in all sectors. Systems engineers to redesign work processes for optimal efficiency will also be needed. For a period, industries will need to train many workers to effectively use new systems to augment their work. In the near term, human workers will continue to be required for most outdoor and physical labor in industries such as mining, construction, forestry, public transportation, and emergency response. Additionally, service industries will continue to require staff to manage employee and customer relationships as public expectations toward work and the purchase of goods and services change (Verhoef et al., 2021). The third decade of the 21st century may be viewed in the future as one of transition, as AI and robotics increasingly augment human work and as the public gains familiarity with automated systems increasingly evident in daily life, whether in shopping, health care, or home automation (Figure 10.2).

Current and Future Trends Affecting Leisure and Play

The lockdowns of the global pandemic of 2020 challenged individuals who had never experienced isolation to become more creative in coping with socially restricted environments. Leisure and play are effective methods in the reduction of perceived stress (e.g., Smallfield & Molitar, 2018; Zhang et al., 2021). Studies document significant reductions in the time and quality of physical, social, and cultural play and leisure participation by children and adults during the pandemic (e.g., Liu et al, 2022; Neville et al., 2022).

Also, during the pandemic of 2020, technology enabled the leisure and hospitality industry to become more creative and flexible after vaccines enabled a broader return to activity. However, even during the pandemic, theme parks and leisure centers found ways to use AI to manage admission, online payment, and capacity to comply with social distancing guidelines. Online trip planning was upgraded to enable coordinated multi-activity scheduling and booking. Some leisure activity businesses also began incorporating gamification, or the addition of video game elements, to enhance their experiences. Augmented reality (AR), where real-time experiences are enhanced by computer driven visual, sound

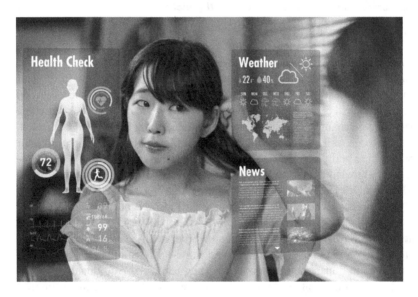

Figure 10.2 The Internet of Things (IoT) will increasingly permeate everyday life. Here, a smart mirror is depicted that provides environmental information, customized news, and personal health data (Metamorworks via iStock, used under license)

and touch sensations, has also been used to enhance leisure experiences. Both AR and VR technologies have evolved rapidly in the past decade and can be expected to continue to be combined with real-time experiences for both leisure and non-leisure purposes in the years ahead (Luck & Aylett, 2000).

Technology, Lifestyle, and Well-being in the 21st Century

The lifestyle-related social determinants of health that were discussed earlier in this book are applicable to this discussion. The 2019 **Global Burden of Disease Study (GBD)** showed clearly that social and demographic factors in developing countries continue to improve overall health (GBD, 2019). But in richer nations, there is a significant mismatch between the chronic health conditions that require health resources (e.g., obesity, blood pressure, diabetes, etc.) and public health spending on efforts to prevent them (Murray et al., 2020). These chronic conditions are not only preventable, but related to lifestyle habits, and can be improved with economic incentives, public education, and public policy. Unfortunately, political and cultural attitudes toward independence and individual freedoms often conflict with public health goals and strategies that can reduce chronic illness.

Beyond excessive use, the adverse health consequences of increased Internet connectivity and AI-driven message targeting have become widely apparent. Misinformation and disinformation strategies have been used as tools to stoke fear and advance political interests within nations and as a medium for propaganda between international adversaries. During the pandemic, there was widespread misinformation being spread on social networking platforms, and some of this false information was associated with public health consequences or violence (Rocha et al., 2023). Health and medicine are topic areas vulnerable to false information because fewer users have the prior knowledge necessary to dispute their validity (Ha et al., 2021). False health information can also be used maliciously as a tool to create societal confusion and fear.

Many countries now have cyber warfare units trained to infiltrate networks and access classified information, or worse yet, disrupt organizational networks and interfere with the operation of critical infrastructure, such as energy grids, air traffic communication, and public transportation systems (Faruk et al., 2022). On an individual level, unauthorized access to personal information through networks can lead to identity theft, extortion, and financial loss if account security is breached. At the population level, stringent security systems powered by AI are commonplace to thwart cybercrime (Ahsan et al., 2022). Such systems, now widespread, are designed to maintain public trust and social capital. However, they can also stoke conflict and raise ethical dilemmas about individual rights and freedoms versus the safety of groups and the greater public good.

Lifestyle Changes Signaled by the General Social Survey

The General Social Survey (GSS) of the United States is a respected biannual survey of changing social attitudes, behaviors, and trends. The GSS is a project of an independent research organization, the National Opinion Research Center (NORC), at the University of Chicago, with principal funding from the National Science Foundation. The GSS is useful for trend analysis because its rigor and recurring core survey items enable generational comparisons (Marsden et al., 2020). The most striking trend data from the GSS pertain to *work, retirement, marriage,* and overall *optimism.*

For the first time in decades, the 2018 GSS revealed less optimism for the future, and diminished expectations for an improved standard of living (Hout, 2020). The GSS also showed that younger cohorts have more accepting attitudes toward marijuana use and sex outside of marriage as well as diminished participation in religion and less agreement with the idea that hard work, rather than luck, leads to success (Hout, 2020). These questioning attitudes extend to marriage as an institution, but also reveal greater openness to the idea of living alone and more tolerance for social diversity, in general. Paradoxically, this tolerance does not extend to older adults, where ageism is globally evident and growing (Marques et al., 2020). This is problematic because ageism is associated with increased isolation and poorer health among older adults (Ayalon et al., 2021). Biased social attitudes toward older adults were particularly apparent during the pandemic of 2020 (Meisner, 2021).

Environmental Stressors and Mental Health

Global political tensions and violence, frequent global weather events, and earthquakes with catastrophic damage have challenged disaster response mechanisms and taxed national economies. Emerging evidence shows that severe weather disasters have a measurable psychological impact on well-being while causing economic hardships (Ahmadiani & Ferreira, 2021). Additionally, wars, natural disasters, and economic disparities have increased migration, often creating political strife where migrants resettle, and leading to negative health consequences (Ellis et al., 2019; Ghosn et al., 2019; see Figure 10.3).

There is some evidence that younger adults, especially college students, have experienced more mental health symptoms (alcohol use, perceived stress, etc.) than other cohorts (Charles et al., 2021), but a widespread presence of these coping problems across cohorts has not been demonstrated. Traffic death data reported by the Department of Transportation shows a decade long high in fatalities, continuing a trend that began after the pandemic lockdowns (Stewart, 2022).

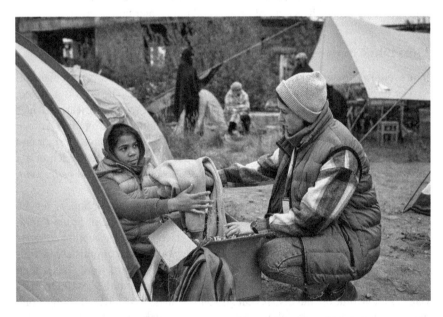

Figure 10.3 Political events, climate change, and natural disasters have led to increasing numbers of refugees. Support for victims includes the provision of mental and physical health services (Shironosov via iStock, used under license)

These data demonstrate a growing trend of fatalities caused by excessive speed, distracted driving, and injuries to pedestrians (U.S. Dept. of Transportation, 2022).

Implications of These trends for Occupational Therapy in the 21st Century

How the trends described in this chapter will affect health care and occupational therapy will likely depend on two key factors: *Economics* and *Technology*. The delivery of health care is already being influenced in wealthier nations through technological advances in communication, diagnosis, intervention, and self-management. Many of these advancements involve the use of dedicated applications on smartphones (Nimkar & Gilles, 2019), an area known as **mHealth** (short for mobile Health). With the evolving capabilities of AI, these advancements will accelerate personalized health care, enabling improved self-monitoring and self-management. However, government attention to mHealth in Germany suggests that realizing the full potential of this technology will depend on regulation, reimbursement structures, and reliable ways to protect personal safety and privacy (Gerke et al., 2020). Also, the success of these mHealth advances will also depend on its demonstrated impact on population health.

A second area that will experience dramatic advancement is that of neuroprosthetics and assistive technologies. The development of sophisticated prostheses having human machine interfaces is transformative and can have a multiplicity of applications. These prosthetics go beyond lower and upper extremity function, to include such advancements as miniature devices to replace the retina (Yu et al., 2020). Functions are controlled by connections between the nervous system of the user and the device through advanced electrodes. The most sophisticated devices for the extremities now under development enable the perception of finely calibrated touch and pressure and the virtual mimicry of pre-injury level movements (Go et al., 2022). Using nanotechnology, advanced sensing devices are envisioned for a wide range of applications (Wang et al., 2020). For each of the technological areas under development, challenges exist in commercialization, standardization, and equitable deployment.

A third important development involves the application of AI and robotics for personal assistant robots, personal monitoring, and on-site assistance for persons with disability and older adults (Kyrarini et al., 2021). For the immediate future, these robots may have limited mobility within spaces but not have the functionality or interactive capability of a humanoid robot. They will most likely be used for visual communication and automated control of some smart home features and assistive technologies. With the growing numbers of aging adults in many nations, greater attention to prevention, lifestyle issues, and the needs of older adults related to chronic disease self-management will be needed.

Occupational therapy has a knowledge base and tradition that is rich in interventions to promote healthy habits and facilitate regular engagement in activities that provide personal meaning. The development of mHealth devices in an occupational therapy context is in its infancy. Improved awareness of the potential uses of AI technologies by occupational therapists and the implications of current trends will be important (Tarricone et al., 2021).

Finally, mention is made of the successful launch of the James Webb Space Telescope (JWST) in December, 2021. In astronomy, the data being collected about the nature of the universe has been described as transformative, already challenging extant theories about the origins of the universe and its size and structure. This development comes at the beginning of a renewed interest in human lunar exploration and the challenges of exploring deep space. Eventually, technology permitting, challenges related to extended periods of travel through space will be overcome. This will require an improved understanding of human occupation in space and strategies for maintaining healthy routines in restricted environments. Occupational scientists have an opportunity to contribute useful research to this effort if they think creatively about relevant scientific questions and potential collaborations in the 21st century.

BOX 10.1 THE POINT IS:

- The 21st century has been influenced by significant global changes, including advanced digital technologies, geopolitical tensions, a pandemic, refugeeism, and climate changes. These factors have affected the nature of work, communication, trust in public institutions, global commerce, and social disparities.
- Changes in work caused by the application of artificial intelligence to robotics are sufficiently transformative to be labeled as the Fourth Industrial Revolution.
- Robotics, including robots, chatbots, and bots, represent a fast-growing category of change that has already affected the global workforce in ways not fully understood. Chatbots and bots are replacing white collar jobs while robots are affecting skilled blue-collar work.
- The implementation of generative AI may have more of an impact on work and lifestyles than any other technology ever introduced. The use of natural language chatbots like ChatGPT are enabling new possibilities in nearly every sphere of work.
- The dark side of emerging AI technologies includes the harmful effects of heavy Internet use on adults and children, growing social inequality caused by uneven access to digital technologies, and malicious uses of new technologies that compromise privacy and provide a powerful avenue for cybercrime and cyberwarfare.

References

Acemoglu, D., & Restrepo, P. (2020). Robots and jobs: Evidence from US labor markets. *Journal of Political Economy, 128*(6), 2188–2244.

Ahmadiani, M., & Ferreira, S. (2021). Well-being effects of extreme weather events in the United States. *Resource and Energy Economics, 64*, 101213.

Ahsan, M., Nygard, K. E., Gomes, R., Chowdhury, M. M., Rifat, N., & Connolly, J. F. (2022). Cybersecurity threats and their mitigation approaches using machine learning—A review. *Journal of Cybersecurity and Privacy, 2*(3), 527–555.

Alaa, M., Zaidan, A. A., Zaidan, B. B., Talal, M., & Kiah, M. L. M. (2017). A review of smart home applications based on Internet of Things. *Journal of Network and Computer Applications, 97*, 48–65.

Aly, H. (2020). Digital transformation, development and productivity in developing countries: Is artificial intelligence a curse or a blessing? *Review of Economics and Political Science, 7*(4), 238–256.

American Psychiatric Association. (2013). *Diagnostic and statistical manual of mental disorders* (5th ed.). https://doi.org/10.1176/appi.books.9780890425596

Ayalon, L., Peisah, C., de Mendonça Lima, C., Verbeek, H., & Rabheru, K. (2021). Ageism and the state of older people with mental conditions during the pandemic and beyond: Manifestations, etiology, consequences, and future directions. *The American Journal of Geriatric Psychiatry, 29*(10), 995–999.

Charles, N. E., Strong, S. J., Burns, L. C., Bullerjahn, M. R., & Serafine, K. M. (2021). Increased mood disorder symptoms, perceived stress, and alcohol use among college students during the COVID-19 pandemic. *Psychiatry Research, 296*, 113706.

Cheng, A. (2021). Covid demand gave Etsy a big boost. Will customers stick around post pandemic? *Forbes* (2-26-21).

Collins, B., Garin, A., Jackson, E., Koustas, D., and Payne, M. (2019). *Is gig work replacing traditional employment? Evidence from two decades of tax returns.* Unpublished paper, IRS SOI Joint Statistical Research Program.

Diplomacy.edu (Diplo- the global consortium) (2020). *The future of meetings.* Report on a virtual conference sponsored by Diplomacy.edu. Accessed on September 6, 2022 from www.diplomacy.edu/topics/future-of-meetings/

Dissing, A. S., Andersen, T. O., Jensen, A. K., Lund, R., & Rod, N. H. (2022). Nighttime smartphone use and changes in mental health and wellbeing among young adults: A longitudinal study based on high-resolution tracking data. *Scientific Reports, 12*(1), 1–9.

Dresp-Langley, B., & Hutt, A. (2022). Digital addiction and sleep. *International Journal of Environmental Research and Public Health, 19*(11), 6910. https://doi.org/10.3390/ijerph19116910

Dupont, P. E., Nelson, B. J., Goldfarb, M., Hannaford, B., Menciassi, A., O'Malley, M. K., Simaan, N., Valdastri, P., & Yang, G. Z. (2021). A decade retrospective of medical robotics research from 2010 to 2020. *Science Robotics, 6*(60), eabi8017.

Eakman, A. M., Schmid, A. A., Henry, K. L., Rolle, N. R., Schelly, C., Pott, C. E., & Burns, J. E. (2017). Restoring effective sleep tranquility (REST): A feasibility and pilot study. *British Journal of Occupational Therapy, 80*(6), 350–360.

Ellis, B. H., Winer, J. P., Murray, K., & Barrett, C. (2019). Understanding the mental health of refugees: Trauma, stress, and the cultural context. In R. Parekh & N. Trinh

(Eds), *The Massachusetts General Hospital textbook on diversity and cultural sensitivity in mental health* (pp. 253–273). Humana Cham.

Faruk, M. J. H., Tahora, S., Tasnim, M., Shahriar, H., & Sakib, N. (2022, May). A review of quantum cybersecurity: Threats, risks and opportunities. In *2022* 1st International Conference *on* AI *in* Cybersecurity (ICAIC) (pp. 1–8). IEEE.

Gerke, S., Minssen, T., & Cohen, G. (2020). Ethical and legal challenges of artificial intelligence-driven healthcare. In K. Bohr & K. Memarzadeh (Eds.), *Artificial intelligence in healthcare* (pp. 295–336). Academic Press.

Ghosn, F., Braithwaite, A., & Chu, T. S. (2019). Violence, displacement, contact, and attitudes toward hosting refugees. *Journal of Peace Research, 56*(1), 118–133.

Global Burden of Disease Collaborative Network. (2019). *Global Burden of Disease Study.* Institute for Health Metrics and Evaluation (IHME), Seattle. www.healthdata .org/gbd

Go, G. T., Lee, Y., Seo, D. G., & Lee, T. W. (2022). Organic neuroelectronics: From neural interfaces to neuroprosthetics. *Advanced Materials, 34*(45), 2201864.

Graetz, G., & Michaels, G. (2017). Is modern technology responsible for jobless recoveries? *American Economic Review, 107*(5), 168–173.

Groumpos, P. P. (2021). A critical historical and scientific overview of all industrial revolutions. *IFAC-PapersOnLine, 54*(13), 464–471.

Ha, L., Andreu Perez, L., & Ray, R. (2021). Mapping recent development in scholarship on fake news and misinformation, 2008 to 2017: Disciplinary contribution, topics, and impact. *American behavioral scientist, 65*(2), 290–315.

Haidt, J., & Allen, N. (2020). Scrutinizing the effects of digital technology on mental health. *Nature, 578,* 226–227.

Harari, N.Y. (2018). *21 Lessons for the 21st Century.* Random House.

Heffler, K. F., Sienko, D. M., Subedi, K., McCann, K. A., & Bennett, D. S. (2020). Association of early-life social and digital media experiences with development of autism spectrum disorder-like symptoms. *JAMA Pediatrics, 174*(7), 690–696.

Hout, M. (2020). *A new compendium of trends in the general social survey, 1972–2018: Period and cohort trends and differences by race, gender, education, urban–rural, and region for 276 repeating items.* GSS Report #64. NORC at the University of Chicago.

Howard, J. (2019). Artificial intelligence: Implications for the future of work. *American of Industrial Medicine, 62*(11), 917–926.

Institute of Electrical and Electronic Engineers (IEEE), (2022). *Adapted from a general definition in an article "What is a robot?"*. Accessed on September 10, 2022 at https:// robots.ieee.org/learn/what-is-a-robot/

Ivie, E. J., Pettitt, A., Moses, L. J., & Allen, N. B. (2020). A meta-analysis of the association between adolescent social media use and depressive symptoms. *Journal of Affective Disorders, 275,* 165–174.

Kane, G. C., Nanda, R., Phillips, A. N., & Copulsky, J. (2021). The Digital Superpowers You Need to Thrive. *MIT Sloan Management Review, 63*(1), 1–6.

Khan, S., Kim, J., Acharya, S., & Kim, W. (2021). Review on the operation of wearable sensors through body heat harvesting based on thermoelectric devices. *Applied Physics Letters,* 118(20), 200501.

Kuntsman, A., & Miyake, E. (2019). The paradox and continuum of digital disengagement: Denaturalising digital sociality and technological connectivity. *Media, Culture & Society, 41*(6), 901–913.

Kyrarini, M., Lygerakis, F., Rajavenkatanarayanan, A., Sevastopoulos, C., Nambiappan, H. R., Chaitanya, K. K., ... & Makedon, F. (2021). A survey of robots in healthcare. *Technologies, 9*(1), 8. https://doi.org/10.3390/technologies9010008

Liu, H. L., Lavender-Stott, E. S., Carotta, C. L., & Garcia, A. S. (2022). Leisure experience and participation and its contribution to stress-related growth amid COVID-19 pandemic. *Leisure Studies, 41*(1), 70–84.

Luck, M., & Aylett, R. (2000) Applying artificial intelligence to virtual reality: Intelligent virtual environments, *Applied Artificial Intelligence, 14*(1), 3–32, https://doi.org/10.1080/088395100117142

Madigan, S., Browne, D., Racine, N., Mori, C., & Tough, S. (2019). Association between screen time and children's performance on a developmental screening test. *JAMA Pediatrics, 173*(3), 244–250.

Marques, S., Mariano, J., Mendonça, J., De Tavernier, W., Hess, M., Naegele, L., Peixeiro, F., & Martins, D. (2020). Determinants of ageism against older adults: A systematic review. *International Journal of Environmental Research and Public Health, 17*(7), 2560. https://doi.org/10.3390/ijerph17072560

Marsden, P. V., Smith, T. W., & Hout, M. (2020). Tracking US social change over a half-century: The general social survey at fifty. *Annual Review of Sociology, 46*(1). https://doi.org/10.1146/annurev-soc-121919-054838

Martinez-Martin, E., del Pobil, A.P. (2018). Personal Robot Assistants for Elderly Care: An Overview. In A. Costa, V. Julian, & P. Novais (Eds.), *Personal assistants: Emerging computational technologies* (pp. 77–91). Intelligent Systems Reference Library, Vol. 132. Springer International. https://doi.org/10.1007/978-3-319-62530-0_5

McLeay, F., Olya, H., Liu, H., Jayawardhena, C., & Dennis, C. (2022). A multi-analytical approach to studying customers motivations to use innovative totally autonomous vehicles. *Technological Forecasting and Social Change, 174*, 121252. https://doi.org/10.1016/j.techfore.2021.121252

Meisner, B. A. (2021). Are you OK, Boomer? Intensification of ageism and intergenerational tensions on social media amid COVID-19. *Leisure Sciences, 43*(1–2), 56–61.

Murray, C. J., Abbafati, C., Abbas, K. M., Abbasi, M., Abbasi-Kangevari, M., Abd-Allah, F., ... & Nagaraja, S. B. (2020). Five insights from the global burden of disease study 2019. *The Lancet, 396* (10258), 1135–1159.

Naisbett, J. (1982). *Megatrends: Ten new directions transforming our lives.* Warner Publishing.

Narayanan, S., Chaniotakis, E., & Antoniou, C. (2020). Shared autonomous vehicle services: A comprehensive review. *Transportation Research Part C: Emerging Technologies, 111*, 255–293.

Neophytou, E., Manwell, L. A., & Eikelboom, R. (2019). Effects of excessive screen time on neurodevelopment, learning, memory, mental health, and neurodegeneration: A scoping review. *International Journal of Mental Health and Addiction, 19*, 724–744.

Neville, R. D., Lakes, K. D., Hopkins, W. G., Tarantino, G., Draper, C. E., Beck, R., & Madigan, S. (2022). Global changes in child and adolescent physical activity during the COVID-19 pandemic: A systematic review and meta-analysis. *JAMA Pediatrics, 176*(9), 886–894.

Nimkar, S., & Gilles, E. E. (2019). Chapter 4. Improving global health with smartphone technology: A decade in review of mHealth initiatives. In Information Resources

Management Association (Ed.), *Multigenerational online behavior and media use: Concepts, Methodologies, tools, and applications (3 volumes)* (pp. 54–75). IGI Global. https://doi.org/10.4018/978-1-5225-7909-0

Oxford Economics. (2019). *How robots change the world. What automation really means for jobs and productivity.* Author. Report downloaded Sept 12, 2022 from https://tinyurl.com/28jsxbw6

Parekh, D., Poddar, N., Rajpurkar, A., Chahal, M., Kumar, N., Joshi, G. P., & Cho, W. (2022). A review on autonomous vehicles: Progress, methods and challenges. *Electronics, 11*(14), 2162.

Peters, S. E., Dennerlein, J. T., Wagner, G. R., & Sorensen, G. (2022). Work and worker health in the post-pandemic world: A public health perspective. *The Lancet Public Health, 7*(2), e188–e194.

Petrosyan, A. (2023). *Internet usage world-wide: Statistics and Facts.* Statista, Online article dated Jan 3. 2023. Downloaded January 27, 2023, from www.statista.com/topics/1145/internet-usage-worldwide/

Pew Research Center (2021). About three-in-ten U.S. adults say they are "almost constantly" online. Online survey report dated March 26, 2021, and writtenby A. Perrin & S. Atske. https://pewrsr.ch/2Y5pwdX

Raj, M., & Seamans, R. (2019). Primer on artificial intelligence and robotics. *Journal of Organization Design, 8*(1), 1–14.

Rocha, Y.M., de Moura, G.A., Desidério, G.A. et al. (2023). The impact of fake news on social media and its influence on health during the COVID-19 pandemic: A systematic review. Journal of Public Health (Berl.) *31*, 1007–1016. https://doi.org/10.1007/s10389-021-01658-z

Schwab, K (2017). *The fourth industrial revolution.* Crown.

Shahrubudin, N., Lee, T. C., & Ramlan, R. J. P. M. (2019). An overview on 3D printing technology: Technological, materials, and applications. *Procedia Manufacturing, 35*, 1286–1296.

Smallfield, S., & Molitor, W. L. (2018). Occupational therapy interventions supporting social participation and leisure engagement for community-dwelling older adults: A systematic review. *The* American Journal of Occupational Therapy, *72*(4), 7204190020p1-7204190020p8.

Smite, D., Moe, N. B., Hildrum, J., Huerta, J. G., & Mendez, D. (2023). Work-from-home is here to stay: Call for flexibility in post-pandemic work policies. *Journal of Systems and Software, 195*, 111552.

Statista (2023). Internet Usage Worldwide. Statistics and Facts. www.statista.com/topics/1145/internet-usage-worldwide/#

Stewart, T. (2022, March). Overview of motor vehicle crashes in 2020 (Report No. DOT HS 813-266). National Highway Traffic Safety Administration.

Tamana, S. K., Ezeugwu, V., Chikuma, J., Lefebvre, D. L., Azad, M. B., Moraes, T. J., ... & Mandhane, P. J. (2019). Screen-time is associated with inattention problems in preschoolers: Results from the CHILD birth cohort study. *PloS One, 14*(4), e0213995

Tan, Z. M., Aggarwal, N., Cowls, J., Morley, J., Taddeo, M., & Floridi, L. (2021). The ethical debate about the gig economy: A review and critical analysis. *Technology in Society, 65*, 101594.

Tarricone, R., Petracca, F., Ciani, O., & Cucciniello, M. (2021). Distinguishing features in the assessment of mHealth apps. *Expert Review of Pharmacoeconomics & Outcomes Research, 21*(4), 521–526.

U.S. Department of Transportation. National Highway Transportation Safety Administration. (2022) Press Release. www.nhtsa.gov/press-releases/early-estimates -traffic-fatalities-first-half-2022.

Vadivu, S. V., & Chupradit, S. (2020). Psychosocial and occupational impact assessment due to internet addiction: A critical review. *Systematic Reviews in Pharmacy, 11*(7), 152–155.

Verhoef, P. C., Broekhuizen, T., Bart, Y., Bhattacharya, A., Dong, J. Q., Fabian, N., & Haenlein, M. (2021). Digital transformation: A multidisciplinary reflection and research agenda. *Journal of Business Research, 122*, 889–901.

Vidal, C., Lhaksampa, T., Miller, L., & Platt, R. (2020). Social media use and depression in adolescents: A scoping review. *International Review of Psychiatry, 32*(3), 235–253.

Wang (2020). Application of zero-dimensional nanomaterials in biosensing. Frontiers in Chemistry, 8, 320. https://doi.org/10.3389/fchem.2020.00320

Young, K. (2015). The Evolution of Internet Addiction Disorder. In C. Montag & M. Reuter (Eds.), *Internet addiction: Studies in neuroscience, psychology and behavioral economics* (pp. 3–17). Springer. https://doi.org/10.1007/978-3-319-07242-5_1

Yu, Z., Liu, J. K., Jia, S., Zhang, Y., Zheng, Y., Tian, Y., & Huang, T. (2020). Toward the next generation of retinal neuroprosthesis: Visual computation with spikes. Engineering, 6(4), 449–461.

Zhang, C., Qing, N., & Zhang, S. (2021). The impact of leisure activities on the mental health of older adults: The mediating effect of social support and perceived stress. *Journal of Healthcare Engineering*, vol. 2021, Article ID 6264447. https://doi.org/10 .1155/2021/6264447

Zheng, P., Xu, X., & Wang, L. (2023) Editorial notes: Industrial Internet-of-Things (IIoT)-enabled digital servitisation. *International Journal of Production Research, 61*(12), 3844–3848. https://doi.org/10.1080/00207543.2023.2202258

Glossary

3D printing   A process for fabricating a physical object from a conceptual model with three dimensions.

Adaptation   A person's development and change in response to challenges. Adaptation may occur at the individual level. The term is also used to describe the process of changing an object or process to fit a contextual circumstance.

Adolf Meyer   The father of American psychiatry and first chairman of the Department of Psychiatry at Johns Hopkins University. Meyer was an early advocate of occupational therapy at its founding and an organizer of the U.S. Mental Hygiene movement.

Affordance   A characteristic in the environment that intuitively invites an action or behavior. An example would be a raised horizontal surface for sitting.

Agency   An individual's capacity to make personal choices and act upon those choices.

Agentic story theme   A life story theme or plot emphasizing personal achievement.

Applied science   A discipline that applies systematic knowledge from a foundational science or sciences. For example, architecture applies foundational knowledge from engineering, and design science.

Archetypal place   A term originated by Spivak (1973) referring to places that meet humankind's basic needs for shelter, space, sleeping, mating, grooming, feeding, toileting, and others.

Artificial intelligence   Complex problem-solving and decisions made by computers and robots that may include speech recognition and language processing, visual identification, navigation, and deep knowledge in defined areas such as medicine or engineering.

Augmented reality   An enhanced interactive version of a real-world environment achieved through digital technology usually involving multiple senses (e.g., vision, sound, touch). May involve holography.

Automaticity   Behavior that is automatic, recurring ,and subconscious.

Automation   The technique of making a device, process or system operate automatically without direct human control.

Basic Rest Activity Cycle (BRAC)   An internal arousal cycle in humans of about 90–100 minutes that influences activity levels.

Belonging   A feeling of fitting in with a group, sometimes viewed as a necessary human need.

Big data   Extremely large sets of data that must be analyzed by computers to be useful. Big data can be structured, unstructured, or semi-structured. Can include video, audio, and text files.

Big Five Model   A conceptual model that describes personality according to one's tendencies across five major traits: Openness, Conscientiousness, Extroversion, Agreeableness, and Neuroticism.

Big Six Model   A conceptual framework derived from John Holland's research that proposes that people can be classified into six major personality types based on their interests. See RIASEC.

Biological domain   A domain of health concerned with structural and functional (physiological) processes that influence health.

Biological rhythms   Internal physiological clocks in humans that influence various functions.

Biopsychosocial Model   An approach, based on general systems theory, that understands health as influenced by biological, psychological, and social factors, as well as the relationships among those.

Bot   A specialized type of robot that uses digital technology powered by artificial intelligence to perform specified functions on the Internet or another network.

Bottom-up approach   A phrase describing an approach to therapeutic reasoning that considers components of function before focusing on occupation.

Chatbot   A specialized type of robot that uses digital technology powered by artificial intelligence to solve problems, make decisions, and produce content through interaction with a human using natural language.

Chronobiology   The study of biological rhythms.

Chronotype   Individual differences related to sleep–wake patterns for activity and alertness in the morning or evening as well as times for peak cognitive and physical performance.

Circadian rhythms   Biological changes that follow a 24-hour cycle. These natural processes respond primarily to light and dark and affect most living things, including animals, plants, and microbes.

Client-Centered practice   A term to describe a therapeutic relationship between a client and provider whereby the client has significant input into goals and therapy, as in a partnership.

Clifford Whittingham Beers   Author of the 1908 best-selling book *A Mind that Found Itself*, and a proponent of the reform of mental asylums. Beers was also an advocate for the mental hygiene movement.

Clinical reasoning   The use of professional knowledge, skills, and reasoning to make decisions in the therapeutic process.

Co-occupation   Shared interactive and responsive doing involving two or more people.

Coherence (in life narrative)   A story with logical order, continuity, and discernable meaning when viewed as a whole.

Communal story   A life story with a theme characterized by or emphasizing social or family relationships.

Competency   The ability to do or act on something successfully.

Conceptualization   Forming an idea or concept about something.

Context   Environmental and person factors that influence the individual and occupational performance.

Core projects   A person's highly valued projects toward which they have commitment because the projects are seen as essential and meaningful in their lives.

Cultural competence   Having the knowledge, practice, attitudes, and skills to serve people from diverse groups.

Culture   The customs, values, practices, and beliefs of a particular social group or nation

Design for all   A design philosophy emphasizing respect for human diversity, social inclusion, and equality.

Desynchronosis   The technical term for jet lag.

Disuse syndrome   A reversible condition caused by sedentary behavior characterized by loss of muscle mass, reduced joint range, sensory symptoms such as tingling and numbness, and reduced endurance. Disuse syndrome can be treated through increased activity and improved nutrition.

Eclecticism   Deriving ideas from many different sources.

Environment   The conditions that surround an individual. These may include physical characteristics, or social and atmospheric conditions.

Environmental press   Environmental factors that influence actions.

Eveningness   A term given to describe the temporal characteristic of people who favor activity in the evening.

Evidence-based practice   Approaches to health care that are supported by rigorous research.

Facet   A sub trait, a component of a general personality trait.

Flow   Term given by psychologist Mihaly Csikszentmihalyi to describe occupations that have an engaging or timeless quality to the doer.

Fourth Industrial Revolution   A designation given to the era from around 1950 to the present during which artificial intelligence and digital technology have created transformative changes in the ways people work and live.

General Social Survey (GSS)   A respected biannual survey of changing social attitudes, behaviors and trends conducted by the National Opinion Research Center associated with the University of Chicago.

General systems theory (GST)   An approach to understanding the concepts and principles behind complex arrangements of related structures that work together to result in an outcome. Credited to Ludwig Von Bertalanffy (1950).

Generative artificial intelligence   An advanced type of artificial intelligence that creates original content based on natural language processing, fast processors, and extremely large volumes of data.

Generative story   A story with a theme featuring help or the mentoring of a younger relative or associate.

Gig economy   Descriptor given to endeavors whereby people earn income by providing on-demand goods or services, sold through digital platforms or websites.

Global burden of disease study   A periodic population health report begun in 1990 by the World Health Organization to provide an overview of the mortality and disability caused by global health conditions.

Goal planning   Setting meaningful and measurable occupation-relevant goals based on the evaluation results and interview with the client and/or caregivers.

Habit   An automatic or recurring behavior or action that is subconsciously performed.

Habituation   A psychological tendency to act in recurring ways.

Herding   The term used for group animal behavior whereby species live in groups and cooperate for survival purposes.

HEXACO Model   A conceptual model of personality that describes personality according to six major trait groups: Humility and Honesty, Emotionality, eXtraversion Agreeableness, Conscientiousness, and Openness to experience.

Identity   The implied central (or first person) figure in a narrative or life story.

Infradian rhythm   A biological rhythm lasting longer than a day.

Institutionalization   Prolonged residence in an institution (e.g., psychiatric facility, jail, or prison).

Interest (psychological)   A consistent or stable preference or attraction toward a subject area, such as music, or science.

Internet addiction disorder   A habit disorder characterized by a compulsive need to spend excessive time on the Internet to the point where it interferes with relationships and other important areas of life.

Internet gaming disorder   A specialized type of addiction or habit disorder characterized by addiction to Internet games.

Internet of Things (IoT)   The networking or connection of devices within everyday objects that can send, receive, and process data through the Internet. For example, a smart thermostat can connect to a phone or a central control through the Internet to manage a home or building environment from distant locations.

Maladaptive   Not adapting satisfactorily to the current situation.

Marginalization   Social exclusion, or the placing of an individual or group at the periphery of a group or society.

Meaning   The subjective interpretation or understanding of a phenomenon or experience.

Meaningful occupation/activity   Meaningful occupation is purposeful human activity that meets basic needs, provides subjectively positive experiences, and contributes to a person's overall assessment of life satisfaction.

Medical model   A reductionistic approach to understanding illness and disease based on the structure and function of the human body.

Mental hygiene movement   A movement started in 1908 to improve care of mentally ill persons as well as to advocate on the social prevention of mental illness through childrearing, adequate work and living conditions, and accessible mental health services.

Meta-analysis   A study of many published studies on the same topic for purposes of determining the consistency of findings and the overall scope of subjects and settings.

mHealth   A general term used to describe the use of mobile technology for health and medical purposes.

Mind–body dualism   An approach to understanding humans proposed by French philosopher and intellectual Rene Descartes. It asserted that there was no connection between the body and mind.

Mixed-methods research   Research examining both quantitative (objective) and qualitative (subjective) variables or factors.

Morningness   A term given to describe the temporal rhythms of people who favor activity in the morning.

Motivation   An influence behind a human action.

Narrative   The academic term for an account or description in storied form.

Non-sanctioned occupations   Occupations viewed as unhealthy, illegal, immoral, or unacceptable within a cultural group.

Occupation   (*n.*) An everyday activity that has individual or shared meaning in the culture. (*v.*) the act of performing or doing a purposeful activity.

Occupation-based evaluation   An evaluation in which the therapist uses an "occupational lens," meaning that the focus is on a person's capacity to do specific daily activities. Often this type of evaluation involves performance of an occupation within the evaluation.

Occupation-based intervention   Occupation-based intervention that uses occupations within the therapeutic process to achieve established goals.

Occupation-focused assessment   Assessment tools that emphasize occupation and assess occupational performance.

Occupation-focused intervention   As defined by Fisher (2014), occupation-focused intervention keeps occupation and occupational concepts at the core of intervention.

Occupational adaptation   Human adaptation to develop mastery in occupational performance.

Occupational apartheid   A term describing social practices and policies whereby occupations are given or denied based on circumstances such as gender, race, nationality, etc.

Occupational being   A term given to describe people from the standpoint of their natural drive to engage in occupations necessary for survival and physical and mental well-being.

Occupational deprivation   Prolonged restriction from engagement in meaningful occupation.

Occupational determinants   Factors, including economics, policies, and social values that may influence occupational participation.

Occupational development   Changes over a lifetime in what people do because of natural maturation, growth, or development.

Occupational disruption   Temporary disruption or change in occupational engagement due to external factors (e.g., time limited illness).

Occupational enablement   Intervention solutions to permit occupational performance.

Occupational engagement   Personal involvement in an activity that involves attention, interest, and purpose; thereby making it meaningful to the doer.

Occupational form   The objective set of physical and sociocultural circumstances external to the person at a particular time.

Occupational imbalance   People spending too much time in one type of occupation at the expense of other necessary occupations.

Occupational injustice   Denial of occupational opportunity that may result from societal rules, injustices, and policies.

Occupational load   Amount of time, intensity, and number of roles and tasks an individual takes on at a time.

Occupational marginalization   Social condition whereby people are denied the opportunity for occupational participation through situations such as policies and practices.

Occupational performance   A person's completion or performance of daily activities.

Occupational justice   Equitable opportunity and resources to engage in occupation.

Occupational perspective of health   A particular view of health from the perspective of humans as occupational beings (Wilcock, 1998).

Occupational profile   Collective information gathered on a client's occupational history, interests, and skills.

Occupational rights   The right of all people to engage in meaningful occupation.

Occupational science   The systematic study of people as doers, sometimes referred to as the science of everyday living.

Occupational therapy   A profession that integrates meaningful occupation as an approach to helping an individual attain, regain, or maintain.health and well-being.

Participation   Taking part in an event or activity.

Participatory Occupational Justice Framework   Occupational justice framework developed by Whiteford and Townsend to enact principles of occupational justice.

Performance capacity   An individual's skills and abilities and their effect on capacity to perform.

PERMA Model   A model of well-being proposed by Martin Seligman that identifies five requisite factors: positive emotions, good relationships, meaning in one's life, a sense of goal accomplishment, and engagement in activity.

Personal projects   A term credited to Brian Little (1983) defined as an inter-related sequence of actions intended to achieve some personal goal.

Personal projects analysis (PPA)   An approach to identifying and studying an individual's current projects to understand their personal-related characteristics, such as their perceived importance, enjoyment, difficulty, etc.

Personality   The combination of characteristics that form a person's distinctive temperament, character, or disposition to behave in certain ways.

Personality trait   A characteristic pattern of behavior, such as being creative or outgoing.

Personality type   The psychological classification of general differences in human behavior. There are multiple theories on personality types. Some of the major types are related to clusters of interests.

Place   A designated location with specific physical or symbolic features or characteristics.

Population health   The general health status of defined groups and populations of people. Sometimes considered a subset of public health, which tends to focus on larger groups.

Practice models   Conceptual tools that provide a guide for how to apply theory to practice.

Psychological domain   A term for the domain of health concerned with thoughts, feelings, and behaviors. Includes personality.

Redemptive story   A story with a theme featuring overcoming adversity or trauma.

Resettlement   Moving a set of individuals from one place to another.

Rest cure   An early approach to healing that prescribed restful living, often in specific locations viewed as suitable for recovery based on their natural features and locations.

RIASEC   An acronym representing the six major types of Holland's model: Realistic, Investigative, Artistic, Social, Enterprising, and Conventional.

Robotics   A branch of technology concerned with designing, constructing, and using artificial intelligence in automated systems to perform complex and specialize human tasks. Robotics includes *robots* that involve physical machines, *bots*, that are software programs that perform electronic functions, and *chatbots*, that are bots which interact with humans using natural language.

Routine   A particular and recurring sequence of tasks or activities.

Salutogenesis   The study of the origins of health and factors that contribute to health and well-being.

Salutogenic   Contributing to health and resilience to disease.

Semiotics   The study of symbols and symbolic meaning.

Sensory deprivation   The absence or removal of stimuli from one or more human senses. Can be environmental or intentional.

Service delivery models   Models of service delivery that may include (but are not limited to), direct service and consultative services that may be delivered to individuals, groups, or populations.

Sleep–wake cycle   A circadian cycle in many living things, including humans, known to be influenced both by daylight and darkness, as well as physiological processes.

Social capital   A concept from the social domain that describes the overall climate of trust and cooperation within groups of people living in the same proximity.

Social cognitive theory   Developed by Albert Bandura, social cognitive theory emphasizes that learning occurs within a social context through interaction with others and the environment.

Sociocultural   Pertaining to factors influencing the differences in social and cultural groups, which may include values, beliefs, habits, and activities in daily life.

Sociocultural niche   Being naturally drawn to occupations because of one's culture.

Social determinants of health   Factors such as living circumstances, economics, and access to education and basic social necessities such as health care.

Social domain   A domain of health concerned with community factors that influence interpersonal relationships between people.

Social jet lag   A chronobiological disorder whereby an individual's biological clocks are not synchronized with their lifestyle, thus disrupting daily routines.

Social Rhythm Metric   A measure of the regularity of daily routines used to detect desynchronosis or jet lag.

Standardized interventions   The use of detailed protocols and manuals to describe how therapeutic interventions should be consistently done.

Stigma   Negative and often unfounded beliefs about a person or group of persons.

Tailored Interventions   Therapeutic approaches that are individually chosen or modified for the personal characteristics of the client.

Temporal adaptation   A conceptual framework advanced by occupational therapy theorist Gary Kielhofner aimed at understanding the role of recurring behaviors such as habits and routines on the occupations in a person's life.

Temporality   The lived experience of time.

Therapeutic use of self   The process whereby the therapist consciously uses the professional relationship with the client to help facilitate therapeutic outcomes.

Time use research   The study of the types and durations of activities by individuals and groups over a 24-hour period.

Top-down approach   Occupation, meaning, and roles are the primary focus of therapy, e.g., using an occupation-based vs. component-based approach.

Ultradian rhythm   Biological cycles that take place within a 24-hour period such as temperature, heartrate, digestion, etc.

Virtual reality   Simulated digital experiences involving realistic 3D displays and human–computer interaction involving movement.

Visitability   Basic design features of houses that allow them to be lived in or visited by persons with mobility challenges.

Volition   Completing something willfully, the motivation for doing something.

Water cure   An early approach to recovery from illness or disease that involved bathing, or water immersion, often in natural hot springs.

Well-being   A positive state that includes a person's state of health and satisfaction with one's current life situation.

Work cure   An early approach to recovery from illness or disease that involved involvement in productive tasks, including work. A precursor to occupational therapy.

Epilogue

This book has offered a beginning guide for understanding how the *doing* of everyday meaningful occupations influences health, well-being, and quality of life. Key concepts about human occupation were identified, and an introduction to applying these concepts in the occupational therapy process was provided. This application of concepts illustrated the interconnections of *person, occupation, environment,* and *occupational performance.* Important factors that influence occupation, such as a person's *culture, worldview,* and fair access to meaningful occupational opportunities (*occupational justice*) were discussed. The competent application of these concepts using occupational therapy theories, models, and frames of reference is fundamental to effective practice. A full understanding of clients and their occupational profiles is a key part of this process.

Having completed the chapters in this book, answers to the following questions should be apparent to the reader:

1. What key concepts should occupational therapists know about occupation?
2. What characteristics of occupations are related to health and well-being?
3. What can personality psychology contribute to the understanding of a client?
4. How are meaningful occupations, identity, and life stories connected?
5. How does occupational science support and enhance occupational therapy (and vice versa)?
6. How is meaning formed by a client and how can a therapist assure that meaning is considered in therapy?
7. What are key considerations when determining the use of a frame of reference, evaluation, or intervention?
8. How does culture influence occupation and occupational therapy?
9. How can therapists ensure principles of occupational justice in the practice of occupational therapy?

10. How are known trends in the 21st century likely to influence the nature of occupation and the types of client problems that occupational therapists may encounter?

Perhaps the most important question is this: *How can occupational therapists apply their expertise in occupation to assure that the full potential of their profession to serve humanity advances confidently into the years ahead?*

Index

Note: Locators in *italic* indicate figures and in **bold** tables

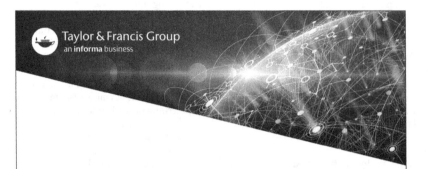

Printed in the United States
by Baker & Taylor Publisher Services